Zero Trends

Health as a Serious Economic Strategy

Dee W. Edington, PhD

Health Management Research Center

University of Michigan

Zero Trends

Health as a Serious Economic Strategy

ISBN Number: 978-0-615-28019-6

Printed in the United States of America

Publisher: Health Management Research Center

Author: Dee W. Edington, PhD

Production and Design: The WorkCare Group, Inc.®

Printed on acid-free, ECF, and SFI certified paper

Distributed in the United States by

Health Management Research Center

University of Michigan

1015 East Huron Street, Ann Arbor, Michigan 48104

Phone: 734.763.2462 • Fax: 734.763.2206

www.hmrc.umich.edu

Zero Trends is an important book for two reasons.

First, it identifies a major problem that must be solved: the rising cost of healthcare in America, which is eroding profits at an accelerating rate and leading toward disaster for businesses, shareholders, and employees. Until something is done about this alarming trend, companies will have to close up shop or make the tough survival decision of no longer providing healthcare for their people.

Second, the book suggests how leaders can reverse this trend in a way that can help us all learn to implement change in the organizations we work in and support. As Dee Edington points out, our do-nothing strategy of the past simply isn't working. Edington doesn't just identify the problem; he also rolls up his sleeves and shows us how to solve it by moving from a sickness-oriented culture to a culture of health, a culture in which we not only care for the sick but also enable the healthy to stay healthy. It's an approach that lowers healthcare costs and at the same time increases productivity and human satisfaction.

Edington clearly spells out the steps to getting this done. To make it work, top management support is imperative and developing a culture of health must become a high priority. The culture of health initiative must be driven from the top and sustained by continual follow up. In life and in organizations, you get what you reinforce. Support and follow up! Support and follow up! Without them, we're just making noise.

Thanks, Dee, for warning us just how grave the pending healthcare disaster is in our country and for pointing us in the right direction to turn it around.

—Ken Blanchard, co-author of *The One Minute Manager*® and *Leading at a Higher Level*

Dedication

This book is dedicated to the memory of Donald E. Vickery, MD (1944-2008), a true pioneer in the field of self-care and demand management. He was all about helping individuals find the tools to allow them to become their own self-leaders in directing the state of their health. He was credited as saying that the key to the future of medicine is shifting its emphasis to wellness. Don was a friend for nearly 20 years, and he always was available to discuss science at any time of the day. His company, Health Decisions International, was an early innovator in health coaching including self-care, disease management, and overall demand management.

I also want to dedicate these writings to my family: Ruth and Everett Edington, who taught me the value of work; my wife, Marilyn, who supported me through several intellectual careers, the final 33 years being in the School of Kinesiology at the University of Michigan; and to David and his wife, Stacie, who are a great source of personal pride as they find the right balance of careers and health in their lives.

Acknowledgements

First, I would like to acknowledge the work of several key individuals, without whose commitment this book never would have seen the light of day. MargaretAnn Cross, who spent hours listening to me talk and created the first set of notes and worked on each of the many drafts over the course of the past two years. In addition, she conducted more than 50 interviews from which she created the stories and quotes throughout the book. Ken Blanchard, who reviewed several of the drafts and provided many valuable suggestions for revisions and offered frequent counseling and encouragement when needed—which was often. Margie Blanchard, who shared many of her learnings as co-founder and President of The Ken Blanchard Companies and as Head of the Office of the Future. Marilyn Edington, who edited many of the drafts, suggested many of the quotes, and contributed much thoughtful advice throughout the creation of this book and during her many years as a colleague in the Health Management Research Center. George Pfeiffer, who offered advice at all levels throughout the process and for his 35 years in this field. Pat Materka, who has known my writings for more than 25 years, for invaluable editing of the final draft and for providing constant encouragement.

Second, a special acknowledgement is due to all those individuals who worked, and those who still work, in the Health Management Research Center at the University of Michigan. They have paid the price over these 30 years as they systematically moved us from a position of identifying the issues to solving the puzzles of the roles of lifestyles, risk factors, and workplace environments as precursors to wellness and to sickness. We hope that through our work, and coupled with the work of others, we have moved to a better place where we can learn to minimize the economic strain in businesses and individuals, and pain and suffering in individuals.

Many individuals volunteered their time through interviews and correspondence to share their experiences through the stories and quotes that are scattered throughout the book. Their contributions allow the book to come alive and I regret not being able to use their interviews in totality—there is so much richness in their stories. So many additional individuals have made major contributions to our thinking and to the words in this book that I regret my space is too limited to name them all.

Finally, I need to acknowledge the more than 400 organizations that invited us to speak to their employees, customers, potential customers, and leadership over these past many years. I only can hope that we helped to create an environment in which they learned as much as we did during those sessions.

Companies throughout the world are beginning to invest in creating
work cultures where promoting wellness and
treating sickness are equal partners.
In some small way I hope this book will add value to that investment.

Table of Contents

Final Words

Executive Summary

"The world we have made as a result of the level of thinking
we have done thus far creates problems we cannot solve
at the same level of thinking at which we created them."
—*Albert Einstein*

Sense of Urgency

This book was written with the sense of urgency and passion I feel on behalf of the people, the business community, our country, and the world. Although I have had this concern for many years, it clearly escalated during the financial meltdown beginning in the fall of 2008. Crises create opportunities, and the current economic crisis demands that companies change the way they do business. In doing so, businesses must realize even more the value of a healthy and productive workforce.

In this book, I often quote Einstein about his notion that the same level of thinking that got us into this situation will not be the level of thinking that will get us out of it. It is clear that after all of these years of the same medical approaches to managing health, more doctors, nurses, hospitals, procedures, and devices will not solve the problems. I respectfully disagree with those in the medical profession and some of the health economists and politicians who argue that prevention and healthy lifestyles will not lower the total costs of sickness or lead to a better way of life for individuals and businesses. The data and information presented in this book will support the argument that improved health status will not only reduce healthcare costs for companies but also increase performance and productivity in the workplace. Even the worst case scenario would be better than the results of the past several decades!

Einstein's message captures the urgency and passion that drives me to write this book. Even after 30 years of research, more than 160 publications, and 400 presentations from the Health Management Research Center, we do not claim to have the total solution for enhancing and maintaining the vitality of the workforce. We continue to design and test our strategies in order to make an airtight business case. However, we feel it is imperative to share our evidence-based recommendations at this time. The survival of many American businesses in the global marketplace depends upon shifting medicine's singular focus of managing sickness to a much more encompassing view of managing health. This is the total value of health and the value of total health management.

No company will be successful in a globally competitive world with anything but healthy and productive people. No individual will achieve his or her fullest potential without believing that staying healthy is just as important as treating sickness.

Lifestyle changes alone will not solve all the problems with healthcare in our companies. But lifestyle changes can significantly lower the demand for medical care, which is where health management comes into the picture. Healthy and productive individuals make positive contributions to companies and society that may far outweigh the savings in disease care. This is one of the lessons I have learned from my work: We need to move from the current "wait-for-sickness" level of thinking to a higher level of thinking by adding a "promotion-of-wellness" component to our overall health management system. We need individuals and companies to share our vision. The U.S. economy can't sustain ever increasing healthcare costs and lower productivity. We have to pursue an alternative.

The cost of waiting for people to get sick far exceeds the cost of helping healthy people stay healthy.

It's Time for a Change

This book is written with leadership in mind. The sickness-related costs are rising faster than new products or services can be sold, or increased efficiencies can be developed, or costs can be shifted to employees, or people can be let go, or businesses can find an off-shore solution. The time is ripe to solve this problem; something has to be done now!

"If we keep doing what we're doing, we're going to keep getting what we're getting."
—*Stephen R. Covey, author*

American business leaders are out of patience with healthcare costs that continue to increase at an astonishing rate with little or no increase in quality. We can and we must change.

- Employers must create environments that encourage their employees to stay well in addition to taking care of them when they are sick.
- Individuals have to take on self-leadership for their own health and seek products and services that will help them maintain it.
- Local, state, and national governments must embrace and act upon the fact that healthy and productive people create a community more economically viable, with a higher quality of life.

Integrating workplace and workforce strategies for health into the corporate culture is a critical part of the solution.

With a combined effort we can create cultures within companies and communities that support healthy and productive individuals.

It is *past* the time when companies:

Wait for individuals to get sick

Pay only for sickness

Now *is* the time for companies to:

Pay attention to their healthy champions

Invest in wellness in addition to paying for sickness

Realize the total value of health to the organization

Encourage the total engagement of the entire workforce

Now *is* the time for health plans to:

Roll an equal investment in wellness into their sickness plans

Now *is* the time for individuals to:

Value and take self-leadership of their personal health

Take action to get better, and the first step is "just don't get worse"

Now *is* the time to get to:

High levels of energy and vitality

Cost trends no more than the rate of inflation

A New Way to Do Healthcare

This book is about a **new model for healthcare** in America. It redefines healthcare as a combination of illness *and wellness* strategies. It is designed to help employers enable employees to become self-leaders in maintaining their energy, vitality, and overall performance.

We must drastically change our singular focus on sickness and sickness prevention to embrace an equal focus on wellness and wellness promotion.

What sets my strategy apart from existing viewpoints is emphasized in the major themes of this book: "help the healthy people stay healthy," "don't get worse," and "create a culture of health." These mantras are meant to create individual winners while promoting the health and economic success of the entire population within the company. To bring this about, we need to create a workplace environment that rewards both individuals and organizations. Key stakeholders cannot wait years to realize a return; they need to realize a level of success quickly and at every level.

My goal is to convince decision makers that helping the healthy people stay healthy is far more rewarding economically, culturally, and personally than simply continuing to feed a self-serving medical care system that waits for people to get sick and then profits from that sickness. The current healthcare system is ineffective and economically dysfunctional.

The current challenge is great, and so is the opportunity for each of us to become self-leaders and stewards of our own health. Embracing this challenge will mean less pain and suffering in ourselves and in our families as well as zero growth in healthcare and disability expenditures.

Treat the sick, but also help the healthy people stay healthy.

It is time to redefine health. It is time for companies to engage their leaders and employees to recognize the real value of health. All of us must adopt a "we can do this" attitude.

"The dogmas of the quiet past are inadequate to the stormy present. The occasion is piled high with difficulty, and we must rise with the occasions. As our case is new, so we must think anew and act anew."

—*Abraham Lincoln*

How the Book is Organized

This book is organized into three primary sections: The Mission, The Business Case, and The Solution. Companies that embrace these concepts will be further rewarded by zero cost trends, increased productivity, advantages in recruitment, and retention of their workforce.

The Mission: Regaining Vitality for Corporate America and for Americans

As Albert Einstein suggests, it is time for a new way of thinking about healthcare and to change the organizational and individual conversations around health. This section previews the essential elements of a new health management system for Americans and concludes with the key concepts that set this book apart. My objective is to set readers on the path to developing a strategy to lower healthcare costs by focusing on the culture of the organization, the health status of the employees, and the message: "Don't get worse."

The Business Case: Health Management as a Serious Business Strategy

The second section highlights our work in developing the business case for integrating an effective wellness component into the traditional employer health benefit model. It critically examines the current "waiting for sickness" strategy embraced by most organizations and proposes a new population-based mode that positions wellness first. The information presented within this section demonstrates the corporate and individual wellness and sickness strategies that have proven to be the most effective in controlling costs and improving overall health.

The Solution: Integrating Health Status into the Company Culture

We build upon five fundamental pillars of an evidence-based strategy designed to integrate health status into the culture of the workplace. The objective is to facilitate high-level health status for all employees, therefore economically benefiting both individuals and their companies. This section does not aim to provide a tool kit of resources, but to share the process. For each pillar I outline four research-based levels of organizational engagement to use in selecting investment strategies and measuring results.

Word of Caution

Poor health is a serious individual, business, and economic threat to our way of life. This serious threat cannot be tolerated and thus we need to act now. Therefore, it requires a serious business and economic strategy to reverse past and current ways of thinking and use of resources. The comments and suggestions in this book may be irritating to some readers. I present them as a challenge to find a new level of thinking to address the threats imposed by a healthcare system that promotes a culture of sickness rather than a culture of health. With this book, I am raising the bar for success and issuing a challenge to those willing to become a champion company.

Some readers may find parts of this book redundant. However, I know that not everyone will read it from front cover to back cover. For those who do, I believe that repetition ensures that if you don't get the message at first glance, you might by the second or third time you see it. This is a workable and critical business strategy.

The Journey and Destination

From when we began the journey:

Finding early adopting companies and collecting the available **data**

Analyzing data and creating **information**

Synthesizing the information and creating **knowledge**

Summarizing knowledge and creating a **solution**

To where we can imagine:

A new way to do health management in America;

Health as a serious business and economic strategy

—Dee W. Edington

Health Management Research Center

University of Michigan

March 2009

The Mission

Regaining Vitality in Corporate America and in Americans

"We must find a way, or we will make one."
—Albert Einstein

Guidelines for Reading This Section

It is time to begin thinking differently about healthcare, and to change the organizational and individual conversations around health: to move away from viewing health as merely the absence of sickness, and to embrace the concept of health management as care for both wellness and sickness.

This section previews the essential elements of a new health management system and concludes with the key concepts that set this book apart. The objective of these three chapters is to commence readers on a journey to develop a strategy to lower healthcare costs and increase productivity by focusing on the culture of the organization, the health status of the employees and the dual messages of "don't get worse" and "help the healthy people stay healthy."

Chapter 1: *Change the Conversation around Health*

*"When it is obvious that the goals cannot be reached,
don't adjust the goals, adjust the action steps."*
—Confucius

From a Focus on Disease and Costs to a Focus on Health and Investment

The United States spends more of its gross domestic product on healthcare than any other nation, yet it is far from leading the world on any other indicator of the health of its citizens. We pay more for healthcare, yet we are less healthy. Dozens of other countries have far better statistics as measured by adult and infant mortality rates and overall health status. This either means that the medical care system is more overpriced and less effective, or that Americans are more prone to sickness than other societies of the world. There may be some truth to both premises, but we believe the former is much more likely to be the source of the problem. The medical system in the United States is designed to wait for people to get sick and then treat the sickest members of the population. It's not that medical professionals are not doing as they are trained; they need to continue caring for those who are ill, but we need to add a wellness strategy to sustain overall health and productivity in our workplaces and workforce.

The cost of health is less than the cost of disease

Michael Parkinson, MD, President of the American Academy of Preventive Medicine, sees that, "The U.S. medical-industrial complex can and will consume every dollar allocated to it until and unless we can debunk two myths: that poor health just 'happens' and that 'someone else' pays or should pay for medical care. Employers increasingly understand that the scientific basis of 'poor health' is rooted primarily in behavioral and environmental factors that they—and other family, educational and community organizations—can impact. Employers know that the consumer/employee/patient/taxpayer actually pays for all medical care. And because they see the *full* cost of poor health, they may have the greatest rationale and clout to design new approaches for attacking unnecessary and preventable morbidity, mortality, and healthcare costs."

Our medical system is misaligned with the health, financial, and productivity needs of our companies. Our current path is not sustainable by any measure, be it health status, sickness, mortality, or financial viability. In fact, the situation is getting worse every year. As Albert Einstein suggests, we need a new way of thinking to solve our problem. We can and we must do better.

"According to the Centers for Medicare and Medicaid Services, about 95 cents of every dollar we spend on healthcare in the United States is spent on treatment, and only five cents on prevention. We need to shift that. Even if we find a way to give access to healthcare to every American, unless we start working on the prevention side, we're never going to have good health among Americans."

—Garry Lindsay, MPH
Director of Business Partnerships
Partnership for Prevention

From one overpass in Ann Arbor, Michigan, you can see a huge and expansive new medical sciences research building on the sprawling University of Michigan medical campus, while the renovated 103-year-old building that houses our Health Management Research Center sits nearby. In many ways, this view captures one of the most poignant truths about the American healthcare system: We capitalize on and invest in sickness and almost completely ignore the opportunity we have to help people stay well.

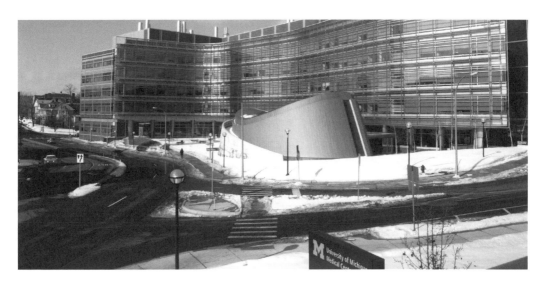

This differential of space raises two key questions.

1. Shouldn't corporations and government focus on promoting healthy environments and wellness care in addition to sickness care?

2. Is helping people stay healthy a worthwhile philosophy and investment for companies and the nation to embrace to improve America's vitality, energy, and competitiveness?

Our answer is obvious.

Our mission is to study lifestyle behaviors and risks and how they impact organizations and influence one's health, productivity, quality of life, energy, and vitality throughout a lifetime.

For years, we have been building the business case for health management. We asked three questions, "What must America change to regain our worldwide competitiveness?" and "Where should we focus our healthcare resources?" and "How can we sustain our workforce as productive and viable?"

The solution, at its core, is relatively simple: Companies and individuals have to change their perceptions and definitions of health from the absence of disease to the presence of energy and vitality.

Change the Conversation around Health and Productivity for Organizations

We need to redefine health. Waiting for people to get sick, and then working to make them better is a failed healthcare strategy. The following five strategies will help move us forward.

Our goal is to change the corporate conversation around health:

1. **From health as the absence of disease to health as vitality and energy**

2. **From only caring for the sick to enabling healthy people to stay healthy**

3. **From the cost of healthcare to the total value of health**

4. **From individual participation to population engagement**

5. **From behavior change to a culture of health**

1. From health as the absence of disease to health as vitality and energy. Organizations can no longer wait until employees and their family members become sick. That approach is like waiting for manufacturing defects to occur and then trying to fix them. The economic and human capital value appears as we start to view health as vitality and energy. Keeping the healthy people healthy adds value on both sides of the economic equation: lower disease costs and increased productivity gains.

2. From caring only for the sick to enabling healthy people to stay healthy. People have not fully committed because we have yet to change the underlying culture. If we follow our historical health-care pattern of only treating one disease after another, we'll continue to suffer, pay, and pay some more, as we have been doing for more than 60 years. Instead of focusing on pulling people out of the river, we have to go upstream and see why individuals are falling into the water in the first place. Then we have to fix those bridges so individuals and families can find safe passages to healthier lifestyles.

Steve Aldana, author of *Culprit and the Cure,* has observed, "As many companies move overseas or south of the border, some are quick to blame free trade for pulling jobs out of America. Jobs are not being pulled out of America, rather constant increases in the cost of healthcare and the dramatic increases in preventable chronic diseases have pushed many companies abroad in an effort to seek lower employee-related costs. Health and wellness programs can help solve both of these problems. Today, the only segment of our economy that has an economic gain from wellness is companies."

We need to build a culture that encourages people to become winners when it comes to health. Corporate and community cultures are beginning to change, and some governments are leading that change by legislating smoke-free environments, increased taxes on addictive products, enforcement of safety belt use, and other measures. Television shows, marketing campaigns, and newspapers are beginning to focus on health in a positive way. Business leaders, health plan executives, benefit consultants, pharmaceutical companies, government representatives, and individuals are talking about the importance of people getting and staying healthy. Employers can make the biggest difference by focusing on the nature of work, job design, supervisory training, ways to recognize and reward employees, and integrating all of these activities into their core values and core way of doing business.

3. From the cost of healthcare to the total value of health. Companies and governments have focused on how much it costs to care for someone who is sick. However, the total value of a person's health is much more than that. It is the sum of the cost of doctor's visits, hospital stays, pharmaceuticals, absences, short-term disabilities, long-term disabilities, workers' compensation, effectiveness while on the job, and a person's impact on others in the organization.

4. **From individual participation to population engagement.** Health promotion or wellness in this country went down the wrong path when the decision was made to focus solely on individuals in specific programs. This strategy typically results in an extremely low participation rate for a wide variety of reasons. Low participation coupled with low success at behavior change results in almost no change in company outcomes. The effective focus needs to shift to programs for populations, which translates, when successful, into total population engagement. Of course programs for individuals will always be in the mix, but they should not be the sole focus.

This was experienced by Don Powell, President and CEO of the American Institute for Preventive Medicine. "When I first got started in this field some 35 years ago, our focus was on personal health management, i.e., helping individuals to change various lifestyle behaviors, such as quitting smoking, losing weight, and managing stress. The results were positive, but somewhat limited in terms of making an economic impact on an organization's healthcare costs. To be more effective, we realized that we needed to reach more individuals.

"This led to our present population health management approach whereby all employees of a company are eligible and encouraged to participate in wellness programs. This strategy has shown itself to be more effective at helping companies reduce healthcare costs and absenteeism as verified in many well designed research studies. We also have realized the importance of offering a variety of delivery options as different people learn in different ways, be it one on one, in groups, through printed material, telephonic coaching, or online. The cliché 'different strokes for different folks' has never been more applicable than in our field."

5. **From behavior change to a culture of health.** Too often and for too long, we have "blamed the victims" because they were too overweight, not physically active, drank too much alcohol, didn't pay attention to cholesterol levels and blood pressure, or took too many drugs. The solution was to sentence them to behavior change programs. Obviously, the individual behavioral change programs have not worked because decades later, more people are overweight, stressed, inactive, hypertensive, and diabetic. Almost none of the risk or disease markers have been improved. Health factors that have changed such as smoking and safety belt use required legislative and environmental strategies to take hold.

"Corporations, the largest sector of our nation, have an inherently vested interest in the health and well-being of their employees. Optimally, this (human capital) is increasingly acknowledged in the causal chain leading from improved individual health, performance, and productivity to profitability in the midst of global competition."

—*Kenneth R. Pelletier, PhD, MD(hc)*
Clinical Professor of Medicine
University of California School of Medicine (UCSF) San Francisco

Change the Conversation to Health and Productivity for Individuals

The root issue is still individual behaviors, and of course this will remain a major part of the success or failure of any strategy. The nation's public health and health promotion goals are not debatable, but the strategies that have been taken to achieve those goals are. Americans essentially have adopted the medical model of focusing on one risk factor or disease at a time. Even though the accepted goals for risk levels, such as the recommended body weight and physical activity level, are correct, they are not realistic. The gap between reality and the goals is too great to bridge in one giant leap of behavioral change. Lasting change occurs in small steps. And there is no guarantee that change, once achieved, is permanent. If a person successfully changes a health risk, but then returns to the environment where it was created, the chances of sustaining the change will be greatly diminished.

Here are three ways to change the individual conversation around health:

1. **Visualize health as energy and vitality, not solely as the absence of disease.**
2. **Believe champions are those who maintain a high health status, with or without an existing disease.**
3. **Embrace a philosophy of "just don't get worse" as the first small step in becoming and staying a winner.**

1. **Define health as energy and vitality, not just the absence of illness.** Americans have to transform their perception of health and embrace its true value. Typically, we think we are healthy if we are not sick or in pain or in the hospital. But health is so much more! Health is having the energy, mobility, and independence we need to live the lives we want to lead, fully, and for as long possible.

2. **Identify role models, the "champions" whose lifestyles put them at low risk for disease and who are vigilant about maintaining their health.** The good news is that many Americans are becoming more conscious of health risks and making healthy lifestyle choices. In fact, it is revolutionary that after years of letting one another engage in unhealthy behaviors, like smoking, drinking excessively, or putting on weight, we're less tolerant of these choices. We are aware of the need to make healthier lifestyle choices ourselves and cheer on the efforts of others making positive change. We admire individuals who become their own self-leaders in this effort. Self-leaders—the champions—deserve to be rewarded through recognition or financial incentives for maintaining their health. This is contrary to the approach of most healthcare professionals and healthcare systems, which is to let people get sick and then rescue them with medical care or disease management.

3. **Embrace a philosophy of "just don't get worse" as the first small step toward improving health.** Individuals need to take a comprehensive approach to becoming self-leaders, and they need to begin with reasonable, achievable goals. The first step is "just don't get worse," which loosely translates as "first, stop the bleeding." As we will show later in this book, not getting worse actually amounts to getting better when compared to the current progression of health risks and disease. This is new and somewhat counterintuitive to the current medical, public health, and health promotion messages, which are silos of information emphasizing increased physical activity, weight loss, smoking cessation, or alcohol reduction. These goals can be achieved over time. "Just don't get worse" is the first step toward getting better.

"*The health of our workforce is inextricably linked to the productivity of our nation's workforce, and therefore to the health of our national economy. It's that central to our nation's viability. We need to address the health crisis in the country, which will then simultaneously address the cost crisis. What can happen is that we can establish a culture of health in which wellness really becomes just a part of doing every day business for an employer, an entire community, an entire state, an entire nation.*"

—Ron Loeppke MD, MPH, FACOEM, FACPM
Executive Vice President, Health and Productivity
Alere

Now is the time to fix our healthcare system, capitalizing on the sense of urgency and need shared by individuals, organizations, and the country as a whole. We must take advantage of this momentum.

Final Word

We have to change, we have to do it together, and we have to do it fast.

Chapter 2: *Health as a Competitive Economic Advantage*

The importance of employers' role in wellness is acknowledged worldwide. The World Health Organization has cited the workplace as one of the priority settings for health promotion in the 21st century.

The Business Need

As a country, we need to redefine health as more than the absence of illness, and to make that concept part of the American culture, we decided to start with the workplace. Many companies for years have offered some form of wellness programming, such as onsite blood pressure checks, weight loss incentives programs, lunch hour fitness walks, and smoking cessation courses. But as well meaning as those strategies are, they have only been marginally successful. The new landscape has to be radically different. Realizing that stand-alone, piecemeal programs aren't sufficient, companies are searching for effective ways to integrate wellness programs into their organizational culture.

There are many large, medium, and small companies that have begun the search for effective strategies. One example is Crown Equipment Corporation, a manufacturing company headquartered in New Bremen, Ohio. President Jim Dicke III believes helping employees and spouses achieve and maintain good health results in healthier employees and a healthier company. Crown invested in this strategy because they believed that the outcomes are supported by research that shows that healthier employees are more productive, have fewer injuries, and have lower medical costs.

> *"With healthier employees, Crown becomes a healthier company and will have a competitive business advantage."*
>
> —*Jim Dicke III*
> *President*
> *Crown Equipment Corporation*

Before expanding the way they do health management, company leaders want proof that the changes will work. However, too little proof exists in the form of longitudinal studies. HMRC's predictive modeling using best practices as the base shows that our recommendation, namely "help the healthy people stay healthy," has a positive impact. Our ongoing studies continue to prove this approach's effectiveness.

A company's main goal is to make money for its owner or shareholders. The good news is that investing in a firm's culture to facilitate a healthy and productive work environment—where employers help employees reduce health risks or maintain their best health status rather than paying only for illness care—is good for the bottom line. It frees illness care dollars to be used in growing the business. Companies must be purposeful and strategic in supporting their employees' health maintenance goals in order to realize these benefits.

Wellness care must gain equal status with sickness care in America.

We dedicated the first two decades of our work to making a business case that employers could use to justify investing in their environment and the health status of employees and their families. In addition, we now know that instituting environmental changes that encourage healthy behaviors works on both sides of the economic equation. That is, an organization or individual investing in health management programs will spend less money on healthcare costs on one side of the economic equation while realizing increased health-related productivity on the other side of the equation. There is no downside! In addition, increased productivity could lead to increased profits or increased reinvestment in the business resulting in more jobs for the local economy. Also more profit leads to increased tax revenue for local, state, and national government units.

Take Rodale Inc., for example, which sees the health of its employees as vital to its success and supports a strong culture of health throughout the organization. Compared to other companies its size, Rodale has lower rates of absenteeism, lower rates of employee turnover, and lower rates of obesity and heart disease. Rodale has had "better than average renewals with our medical/prescription plans" over the past five years. Most companies are missing an opportunity because they are primarily focused on how to reduce or eliminate medical plan expenses," says Amy Plasha, Vice President of Compensation and Benefits. "The bulk of medical and prescription costs are not a result of extended hospital stays or severe critical illnesses. In addition, since these expenses are not those that typically can be avoided or reduced by a specific program or plan design, we have been focused on providing alternative coverage and programs that create a better work-life balance as a means to tackle the most common expenses that our employees face. What they need are things to help them live healthier lives every day, and for the most part, the cost of providing that help is much less than your standard medical expense."

"Managing heath care costs and benefits is not easy in these tough economic times; but retaining top talent should be a high strategic initiative for any company to survive in this global environment. Don't let employees be the blunt of all cost savings; companies should examine all spending before impacting employees. You simply can't win without talent; employees are an investment for the future."

—Michael Bruno
Executive Vice President and CAO
Rodale Inc.

There's no alternative to healthy and productive workplaces and healthy and productive employees if we are to remain competitive in today's global marketplace. Think about this fact: Our American lifestyle—as well as today's workplace and community environments—leads to higher health risks, higher probabilities of disease, and higher costs for sickness care. Everyone needs to recognize this. We see many hopeful trends, and we have seen the changes that can occur with smoke-free environments, limits on trans fats, walking trails, flexible working hours, and work-from-home options, all brought about by visionary leaders. As knowledgeable citizens and responsible companies, we can't miss this opportunity to impact the culture of our workplaces. Unless we integrate a culture of health into the way we do business, we will lose our competitive advantage and our highly valued way of life.

Final Word

No company will be successful in the global marketplace
without healthy and productive people.
If we don't do it, someone else in the world will do it
and our competitive advantage and our way of life will be lost.

Chapter 3: *Create Winners, One Small Win at a Time*

"If you can't explain it simply, you don't understand it well enough."
—*Albert Einstein*

Develop a Sense of Self-Leadership

People like to be part of a winning team, and they want to know that they can succeed. Health is one of the most important ways we define a successful life. A simple but effective chart we use in talking about personal health management illustrates where people with varying levels of risk factors fall on a health continuum. It shows sickness and disease at one end of the continuum and health and wellness at the other (see **Figure 2**). When we show this in a presentation, the first question we ask is, "Where do you want to be on this continuum?" Everyone wants to be near the health and wellness end, and they want to be on one of the arrows pointing in that direction. Then we ask the second question. "Who is the leader who is going to get you there?" Everyone gets that one; if not right away, then after they've had a few seconds to think about it.

These are two very powerful questions. And when people answer them, they understand immediately that they alone are the self-leaders who are going to achieve their wellness goals. We simply have to provide the education and resources they need—and then get out of their way. Self-leaders learn what they need in their lives. They identify their own barriers, and seek out resources to overcome them. Then they implement a plan for personal long-term health and wellness. Later in the third section, we will emphasize the role health coaches can play in helping individuals become their own self-leaders, pointing them to resources available within companies, civic groups, faith groups, schools, social organizations, and communities. Ultimately, the self-leaders turn into the individuals we call "the champions." These winners become role models within the population, and start to recruit other self-leaders by their own example and actions.

Figure 2. Health Continuum for Individuals or for a Population

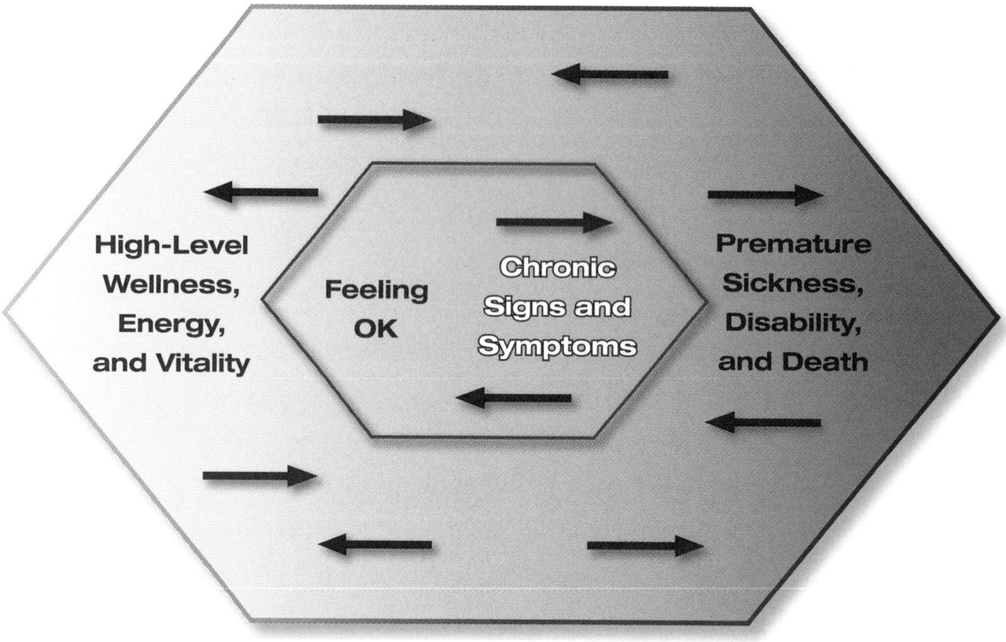

Edington. *CFR.* 2:44, 1983

*"It sounds pedestrian to say it, but the whole idea that it is our job to take care of ourselves—
on our behalf and on everybody else's behalf—has been a revolution."*

—*Helen Darling*
President
National Business Group on Health

Another significant outcome is that in answering the two questions, people realize that while they all want to be on the arrows pointing toward wellness, the American healthcare system is completely based around the arrows pointing toward sickness. Our doctors, nurses, and health systems treat people only *after* they get sick.

One reason is that this is the way medicine has developed over time, but another explanation is that the medical community has tied their economic models *only* to making money when people are sick. There is certainly a strong advocacy for "waiting for sickness" and then charging for treatment.

Which Way Are You Moving?

The good news is, the wellness-sickness continuum illustrates the amazing opportunity to reverse that mistake and move the population in the direction of wellness. Until now, the medical community has invested nearly all of its time and resources in attempting to slow down sickness directed movement, paying the most attention to patients at the far end of the sickness side. The bottom line is that a vast majority of the people want to be on the arrows pointing toward wellness. Perhaps someone should now start paying attention to the desires of the people.

We have to expand what is now an extremely limited focus on the wellness direction. Even the recent emphasis on preventive services tends to emphasize averting sickness rather than promoting high-level wellness. Preventive services are a step in the right direction since they target the high-risk population who do not have a disease, or are still in the early stages of disease. But true success in creating a healthy worksite comes from turning our attention to the wellness-pointing arrows.

"The great thing in the world is not so much where we stand, as in what direction we are moving."
—*Oliver Wendell Holmes*

Creating Winners: It Begins with "Don't Get Worse"

Whether you are an executive running a company that is losing money, an employee who's been diagnosed as pre-diabetic, or a hospital patient losing blood, the first step is always to stop the threat; that is, **just don't get any worse**. You need to halt the downward spiral, take time to recover, and start moving in a positive direction.

Often, one of the first phases of any worksite wellness program is to offer a health risk appraisal to all employees. If we want to make a positive impact on an employee population, 85 to 95 percent of that group needs to know about their risk factors and be willing to say, "That's enough. I am not going to get any worse." Eventually, if appropriate, they need to be asking, "How can I make small improvements and get on the way to recovery?" This is the way we create self-leaders taking responsibility for their health. The goals must be attainable. Each individual has to believe they can succeed.

"We know that someone who has a body mass index of 30 is probably not going to make it down to a body mass index of 25, but we are going to encourage them to maintain their health status or to drop it down to a BMI of 29. And that to us is success. We are moving them in the right direction and we are keeping them from getting worse. Our goal is to try to help each individual be healthy."

—J. Brent Pawlecki, MD
Corporate Medical Director
Pitney Bowes, Inc.

Start with Small Wins

First example: Every hand goes up when we ask an audience, "Can you commit to walking at least 500 or 1,000 more steps a day for the next six months? Can you convince the rest of your company to do this?" We get a different response when we ask about doing 10,000 steps a day (approximately four miles or 1.5 hours) each day for the next six months, which is the goal most often touted by health experts and the media. That's an awful lot of walking for a nation whose population is more prone to sitting and driving than to walking. See Table 1 on page 31.

Second example: "Do you think you and everyone in your company can maintain your current weight for the next six months?" Absolutely every hand goes up. But they're very pessimistic when we ask about losing pounds or achieving a body mass index of 25 in the same time frame.

Third example: People readily agree that they and others in their family, company, or community could check their blood pressure and cholesterol levels, and learn the meaning of the numbers. But they seriously doubt their ability within six months time to lower these numbers or bring them under control.

The point is, contrary to the idealism of the public health establishment, we have to start with realistic goals. If you want to move a population in a positive direction, you have to start with small wins. Public health has actually convinced us that we are losers and failures by setting the initial standards too high for the current American lifestyle. We can create a winning mindset by simply shifting the emphasis to not getting worse as the first step. Our data confirms this fact. So let's start there. Let's create a nation of winners, one step at a time. Once we start winning, the momentum will spur more success.

Table 1. Create "Winners" Health Strategy

The First Step Is "Don't Get Worse"...for Six Months		
Health Status	*The Winner's Strategy*	*The Failed Strategy*
Body Weight	Don't Gain Weight	Reduce Weight to 25 BMI
Physical Activity	Walk 500 Steps/Day	Walk 10,000 Steps/Day
Blood Pressure	Know Your Numbers	Control Your Numbers
Cholesterol	Know Your Numbers	Control Your Numbers
The Second Step is to "Raise the Bar in Small Intervals"		

What About the Workplace Environment?

In the decades between the 1970s and 2000s, public health and wellness professionals made another mistake in interpreting the wellness-sickness continuum. They thought wellness applied only to individuals, and they believed that people's behaviors were causing high healthcare costs. The solutions they proposed centered around behavioral change. As stand-alone programs such as smoking cessation or weight loss, these efforts proved to be relatively ineffective. Even if health counselors convinced people to make changes, they tended to revert to their unhealthy habits after they went back into their unchanged environments.

We now know that we can't just blame individuals. If we want them to become true self-leaders, we must create social and physical environments to enable individuals, families, employees and citizens to succeed. The way to keep healthy people healthy is to first create a facilitating environment and then provide resources for people to change the behaviors that threaten their health.

Look at the changes in American smoking habits, even though it took 50 years to change the image of cigarettes from something fashionable to undesirable and dangerous. Education and higher taxes helped, as did the new laws that address the environment. Because it is now outlawed in many public places, smoking has become as inconvenient as it is unhealthy.

It is clear that individuals won't get or stay healthy by reading a book, by working through a Web site, or taking a health class. They need the support of a healthy environment that rewards their efforts and makes them feel like winners. The healthy environment or culture starts with obvious things like safe, well-lit stairwells, and vending machines and cafeterias that offer healthy food choices. It progresses to flexible job design, comprehensive health benefit design, recognition, rewards, clear career paths, social networks, and more. Of course all of this proceeds from a clear vision from senior leadership and support throughout the company.

"Employers excel at solving problems and turning them into opportunities. That is what business exists to do. So businesses have to stay in the health arena. These are population-based problems, and businesses are very good at creating systems and managing populations."

—*Sean Sullivan*
President and CEO
Institute of Health and Productivity Management

At Crown Equipment Corporation, health management programming began with an emphasis on worker safety and evolved into a full court press toward helping employees reach and maintain the highest level of health and well-being as possible. The company, which has a more than 90 percent engagement rate in its health management programs, offers employees and their spouses incentives to take advantage of health risk assessments, health screenings, health advising services, and a variety of health maintenance and risk reduction programs. One of the biggest achievements has been changing the culture of the organization, says James R. Heap, MD, the company's medical director.

For example, the company used to provide free soft drinks during the break times. Now, employees get a choice of healthier fare—juice, milk, fruit, and baked chips are stocked in free vending machines. "Why would we pay for somebody to drink soda pop, which is not very healthy?" Heap asks. "Now we have health-based criteria for what we offer. That's a major cultural change."

The company also has redesigned its benefit programs to encourage the use of preventive services such as mammograms, pap smears, colonoscopy, and recommended blood tests. "A healthy culture is a number of things," Heap explains.

All of the effort has paid off. In just three years, the number of low-risk employees at Crown has risen from 46 percent of employees to 58 percent, while the employees at a high-risk status dropped from 22 percent to 13 percent. "That's a significant improvement, and it's been a consistent and ongoing change," Heap says.

Summary

Companies can sell more products, raise prices, work harder, work more efficiently, or cut staff in order to pay for more sickness care this year. Where do the resources come from for the next year, and the next? Of course, these strategies may work in the short run, but they are not sustainable in an era of global competition and economic challenge. We have to stop getting worse, or we'll find ourselves bankrupt as individuals, companies, communities, and as a nation.

The challenge is to create environmental change that enables healthy people to stay healthy and encourages those who need to change to do so. We will achieve that only by engaging individuals, families, companies—and ultimately—communities, states, and the nation. We need a universal culture that places high value on sustainable good health.

The good news is that we can now measure the consequences of doing nothing and the benefits of the new health strategy. The data, information, and knowledge we and our colleagues around the world have gathered over the last 30 years have provided the business case for a new health strategy, including helping the healthy people stay healthy. It is imperative to put wellness care on an equal footing with sickness care. In the book's third section, we outline implementation strategies that companies can use to make health an integral part of their core business and worksite culture to create workplace and individual winners.

Final Word

We believe America is on the threshold of great change. Many companies are listening to the message and are ready to help themselves, their employees, and their families and communities maintain or regain energy and vitality.

The Business Case

Health Management as a Serious Business Strategy

"In the middle of difficulty lies opportunity."
—*Albert Einstein*

Guidelines for Reading This Section

The purpose of this section is to highlight our work in developing the business case for adding an effective wellness component to the traditional sickness-based corporate health solution. The first step was to discover the natural flow of risks and costs of a working population. We then can use these natural flows as the basis of an intervention strategy and as evaluation and program feedback for an improved workplace culture and health status in individuals. The data demonstrate that the current "waiting for sickness" strategy is unsustainable in terms of the health status of Americans and in the rapidly escalating healthcare costs without any improvement in quality outcomes. The positive news is that the data demonstrate that changes in health status correlate with changes in costs; however, corporate and individual wellness strategies have proven to be of limited effectiveness in improving overall health status, improving productivity, and lowering healthcare costs. The final chapter in this section demonstrates that "just not getting worse" is the first step toward getting better. The inference from our data is that there is an opportunity for companies to create a health management solution to integrate the wellness and sickness strategies.

Chapter 4: *Waiting for Sickness Is an Unsustainable and Failed Strategy*

*"Insanity: When you continue to do the same thing and get the same
unsatisfactory results."*

—*Albert Einstein*

The Do-Nothing Strategy: Waiting for Sickness and Then Paying and Paying

Consider this: In many communities, the largest employers are hospitals and some of the highest-paid professionals are physicians. Their success depends upon full occupancy of hospital beds, operating rooms, and clinics. The healthcare system has no economic incentive to help people avoid illness. It's to their advantage to wait for sickness to strike and then make money by treating it. This has gone on for decades. Even medical and pharmaceutical researchers are focused on treatments and cures, not prevention.

"Our nation's healthcare system is poised for restructuring of some sort. No matter what direction the overall national strategy takes, policy change is critical to business survival and to each person's individual health status," says Marilyn Pearce Edington, an 20-year colleague in the HMRC before retirement.

"Helping the healthy people stay healthy as a major cost containment strategy is a seismic shift. The focus moves from merely providing care for the sick and diseased to profiting with attention and care for the well," says Pearce Edington. "The Center's data show that such a shift at the worksite will foster greater sustainability and a strong economic return for business and will promote a transformation in the way people embrace their personal health."

And who pays for the disease care system? Companies and individuals! This is a bad deal all the way around for America in terms of cost/benefit. It is ironic that Americans highly value sickness care and, in fact, would accept the high cost if the treatments were the best in the world. But as we pointed out earlier, the U.S. is only near the top in terms of costs and nowhere near the top in terms of medical outcomes.

As we contemplate a solution to the country's healthcare crisis, we must ask the question, "What got us into this mess?" Again, it's the "do nothing" approach: wait until people get sick and then find a way to help—a route that is typically very expensive.

During the late 1990s and the 2000s, the proposed solution to high healthcare costs was exclusively related to access to care and changing the formulas around "who pays." Unfortunately they are still the central focus of most of the proposed healthcare reform plans. Obviously, these solutions were generated at the same level of thinking that got us into the healthcare crisis in the first place. As Einstein suggests, we need a transformational approach based on a new level of thinking. It is clear that more doctors, more nurses, or more hospitals will not solve our current healthcare problems. We must give individuals and corporations the opportunities to become self-leaders, who place a high value on excellent health.

> *"Cure people's ills and make them healthy for a day.*
> *Teach them to stay well and keep them healthy for a lifetime."*
> —*Chinese Proverb*

What Is Driving Our Escalating Healthcare Costs?

Companies always seem to ask, "What is driving our healthcare costs?" Now there is a trivial question! And then they pay consultants a lot of money to come back with the obvious answer: disease! The more interesting question is, "What drives disease?" The answer is, to a great extent, risk factors. We end up focusing on the health risks and behaviors of individuals as well as on unhealthy workplace and community environments. Individuals with high risks often migrate to having disease and high costs, which drive the economic outcomes listed within the box in **Figure 3.** Risk factors

Figure 3. The Economics of Health Status

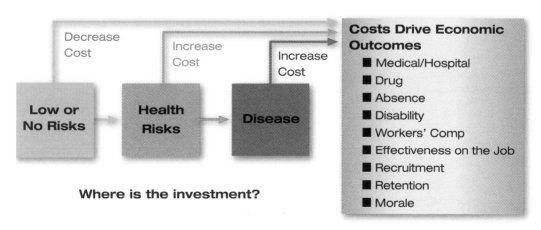

in individuals are characteristics that can be modified, nearly always with much less cost compared to waiting for sickness and then attempting to treat the disease.

One of the root causes of unsustainable growth in healthcare costs is the natural flow of individuals from low risk to high risk to disease to high cost.

Table 2. **Estimated Health Problems**

Self-Reported Health Problems	Percentage of the Population
Allergies	33.2%
Back Pain	26.9%
Cholesterol	16.2%
Heart Burn/Acid Reflux	15.2%
Blood Pressure	14.5%
Arthritis	14.5%
Depression	10.7%
Migraine Headaches	9.4%
Asthma	7.0%
Chronic Pain	6.4%
Diabetes	3.8%
Heart Problems	3.3%
Osteoporosis	1.8%
Bronchitis/Emphysema	1.7%
Cancer	1.3%
Past Stroke	0.7%
Zero Medical Conditions	31.9%

Estimates are based on the age-gender distribution of a specific corporate employee population

From the UM-HMRC Medical Economics Report

Table 2 shows the prevalence of existing disease and risk factors in a working population. Note that the top six diseases are not the ones that are typically expensive in terms of medical and pharmacy costs but they do impact quality of life and productivity on a daily basis. The prevalence of these health risks and behaviors could lead to disease or pain and suffering. Their importance becomes increasingly apparent as we demonstrate the consequences of the do-nothing health strategies.

The prevalence of disease and/or risk factors shown in Table 2 is scary but real. We find similar frequencies in every workforce we survey. If we do nothing, we know that these conditions will naturally progress to the next more complicated and costly level. This unnecessary progression in the direction of more risks and disease will continue to put increasing economic strain on individuals, companies and communities. This situation is the root cause of increasing healthcare costs and decreasing productivity in the workplace and workforce.

The Natural Flow of Health Risks and Costs

Health risks are some of the factors that move people to the left or to the right on the illness-wellness continuum (see Figure 2 on page 28). With disability and early death at one end of the continuum and health and vitality on the other, the choices people make in terms of how they live their lives determine where they are on the continuum and, more importantly, which direction they are heading. Most individuals easily grasp the notion that some activities move you toward sickness, and early disease and disability, while others move you toward vitality, energy, and independence. One of the interesting things about this continuum is that people seem well aware of what it is like to be in the sickness zone but less conscious of what it is like to be in the wellness zone. It is critical to raise awareness on this point if we are to be successful in moving workplaces and workforces into this zone.

One of the tools we use to raise health awareness and determine health risk status in a population setting is through the completion of a health risk appraisal (HRA). The health risks and cut-off points from the HRA are shown in Table 3 (on page 40). The most common and straightforward risk stratification is low-risk status (zero to two of the risk factors), medium-risk status (three to four of the risk factors), and high-risk status (five or more of the risk factors). Many people are surprised to learn that it is the cumulative effect of health risks—not any one risk in particular—that impacts their progression toward disease and high healthcare costs.

The HMRC has processed more than 4 million HRAs from several hundred companies over the past three decades. Many people have completed it multiple times, and in the process, effectively tracked the direction they are moving on the health continuum. The questionnaire provides baseline information to individuals and an overall status report to companies.

A typical company might have 64 percent of employees at low-risk status, 26 percent at medium-risk status, and 10 percent at high-risk status. If the company doesn't do anything to help employees stay well or improve their health status, within two to three years the distribution will be something like 61 percent low-risk status, 27 percent medium-risk status, and 12 percent high-risk status. This underscores the hazard of doing nothing.

The diagram in Figure 4 (on page 42) shows a company's first-year HRA results in the upper rectangle in each of the three health risk status areas. The lower rectangle shows the risk percentages at the end of two to three years. The numbers in the rectangles are interesting but don't tell us anything about where the individuals went during those years. The numbers and percentages associated with the arrows indicate how many individuals or what percent of that risk population moved in

Table 3. **Estimated Health Risks in an Employed Population**

Health Risk Measure	High Risk	High Risk Criteria
Body Weight	41.8%	BMI >27.5
Stress	31.8%	High
Safety Belt Usage	28.6%	Using safety belt <100% of the time
Physical Activity	23.3%	<One time per week
Blood Pressure	22.8%	Systolic >139 or Diastolic >89 mmHg
Life Satisfaction	22.4%	Partly or not satisfied
Smoking	14.4%	Current smoker
Perception of Health	13.7%	Fair or poor
Illness Days	10.9%	>5 days last year
Existing Medical Problem	9.2%	Heart disease, cancer, diabetes, stroke
Cholesterol	8.3%	>239 mg/dl
Alcohol	2.9%	More than 14 drinks/week
Zero Risk	14.0%	

OVERALL RISK LEVELS		OVERALL RISK LEVELS	
Low Risk	55.3%	Low Risk	0 to 2 high risks
Medium Risk	27.7%	Medium Risk	3 to 4 high risk
High Risk	17.0%	High Risk	5 or more high risks

From the UM-HMRC Medical Economics Report

the direction of the arrow over those three years. The transition of individuals is the most important learning and is what we have labeled the natural flow of health risks in our society.

The diagram represents a Markov chain analysis, a mathematical technique to examine longitudinal data from the same individuals, named after its discoverer. Based on these longitudinal data one can solve the equations to find the best strategy to get the most people to low health-risk status. By solving the equations or by just looking at the figure, it becomes obvious that the best solution is to stop the upward flow of people—or simply put, "don't get worse"—and to keep the low-risk people low risk. We must stop the upward migration.

"For individuals who are already healthy, you simply have to provide the resources and make sure they feel that the company supports the use of these programs and services because they will use them, and they'll stay healthy. Your healthy people are your market share.
It's important to keep those people well."

—*Andrew Scibelli*
Manager of Employee Health & Well-Being
Florida Power & Light Company

Most health management professionals pay little notice to the people moving from one rectangle to another. Their first instinct has always been to address only the numbers in the rectangles and to devise ways to improve the health of the medium- and high-risk employees. Many companies initiated their wellness programs with these instincts and remain stuck with this strategy, targeting most of their health and disease management programs at these individuals regardless of where the individuals came from or where they are going.

Our experience is that most often, these single-focused risk-reduction programs do not work for a variety of reasons. In some cases it's the quality of the programs, but more often it's the outcome. Because, even if the programs are successful (and most often they are not successful), even as a few workers move out of the high- or medium-risk category, others are moving in (see the upward arrows in **Figure 4** (on page 42). So if your strategy is exclusively toward reducing high risk, the best you can hope for is just breaking even. Even that outcome is unlikely, since people often revert to their old habits once they return to an unchanged environment. Single, targeted, stand-alone programs simply don't give sustainable results.

A Different Way of Thinking

A more creative way of thinking would be to follow the mathematical solution and stop the upward flow from low risk to medium risk and from medium risk to high risk. The first step is changing the workplace environment and convincing the people in it to adopt the mantra, "don't get worse." These two strategies are key to making health an integral part of the corporate culture. Once people succeed at maintaining their health status, they can take steps to improve it, if needed. A cultural change that is led from the top and embraced by the workforce can score significant gains for individuals and the company.

Figure 4. Natural Flow of Risk Transitions

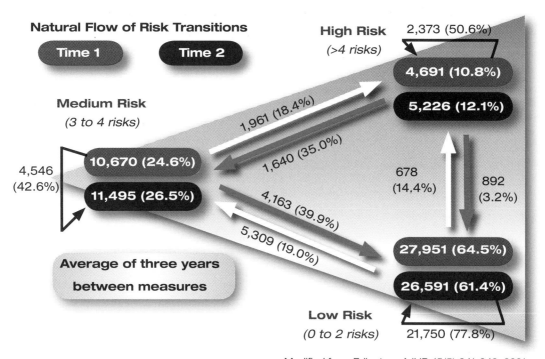

Modified from Edington, *AJHP.* 15(5):341–349, 2001

"It's very difficult to bring someone from an unhealthy risk score to a healthy risk score. It's much easier to keep someone healthy."

—*J. Brent Pawlecki, MD*
Corporate Medical Director
Pitney Bowes Inc.

Our current healthcare and health promotion system pays very little attention to the low-risk category. We simply wait for people to move into higher-risk or disease status, and then we spend a lot of money trying to move them back down. It is far more cost-effective to keep low-risk individuals at low risk. The low-risk individuals are the champions of the population, and we have to create a culture that helps them maintain their champion status.

"Every person you help stay in that low-risk category is a win."
—Amy Schultz, MD, MPH
Director of Prevention and Community Health
Allegiance Health

The Natural Pattern of the Cost of Medical Care

The opportunity to intervene early also emerges by mapping patterns of healthcare risks and costs. Using the HMRC's database, we plotted the flow of costs before and after a high-cost event, such as a heart attack or any very expensive medical crisis. We began by identifying people with healthcare expenses of more than $5,000 in a single three-month period; we then looked at costs for the three years prior to the event and for the three years that followed. Figure 5 (on page 44) also shows the same time frames for people who experienced costs of $500 to $5,000 in a single quarter with those whose costs were less than $500 in the quarter. It's important to note that when an individual experiences a high-cost health crisis, their costs spike due to inpatient hospital costs, but later their overall costs continue to be higher than others. However, in the period before a high-cost event, there's a clear opportunity to identify risk factors and potentially defer or prevent the high-cost episode.

Each person in every population is on one of the three lines in Figure 5. In 70 to 85 percent of all cases, the HMRC can identify three years ahead of time which line people are most likely to be on, just by studying the risks and costs identified on their HRAs and claims data. Diseases often evolve slowly, day by day, risk factor by risk factor. If risks and costs are known a few years ahead of time, we could intervene and possibly avert the crisis.

The 80-20 rule holds true. In healthcare, at any one moment in time, 20 percent of the people cause 80 percent of the costs. The trouble is, by the time you identify that 20 percent, the people have changed and the next 20 percent are knocking at the door. The solution is to get out in front of the cost curve.

Much attention has been focused on projecting an individual's trajectory toward the spiked high-cost individual, and this is clearly one of the major objectives of our work over the past ten years. Now we have the algorithms to be able to put people in a category whereas 75 to 85 percent of the

Figure 5. **Total Medical and Pharmacy Costs Paid by Quarter for Three Groups**

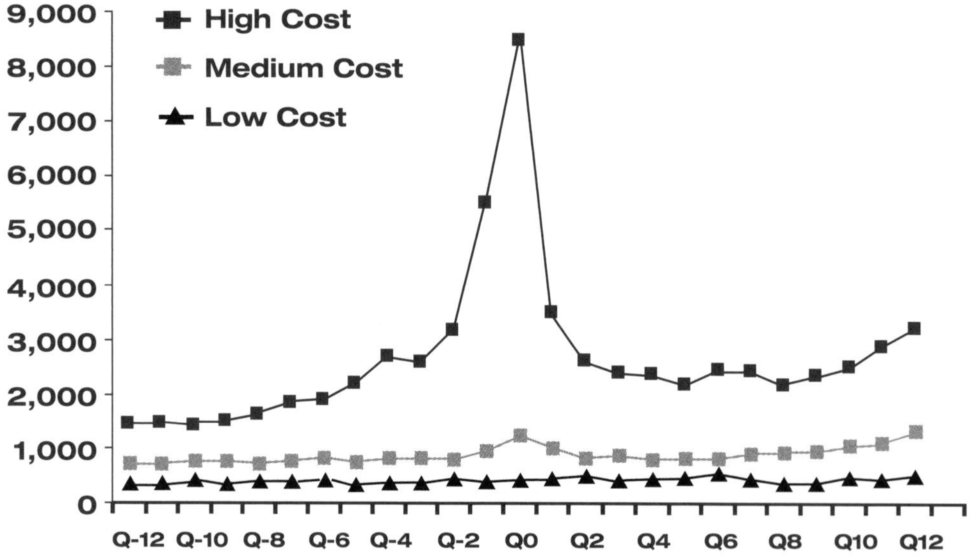

Musich, Schultz, Burton, Edington. *DM&HO*. 12(5):299-326,2004.

time we are correct when we say they are going to be in that high-cost group within the next two to three years. However, we and others need to invest an equal effort into finding the correct algorithms to understand how to project an individual's path toward the low-cost category (less than $500 per quarter). Our prediction, which has already proven true in several studies, is that it is easier to support and maintain individuals on the low-cost path than trying to move individuals off the high-cost trajectory. However, both efforts are necessary to achieve the highest health status possible at any one time. We insist on both tactics.

Age, Health Status, and Costs

Another comprehensive look at the relationship between health risks and healthcare costs appears in **Figure 6** (on page 45). Each individual is represented on one of the vertical bars, according to age and health risk status. Health risk status is determined by risk categories: low risk is zero to two risks, medium risk is three to four risks, and high risk is five or more risks. As **Figure 6** clearly indicates, costs go up as people age, regardless of their health risk status. Also, as health risk status gets worse, costs go up regardless of age.

Figure 6. **Costs Associated with Risks** (*Medical Paid Amount x Age x Risk*)

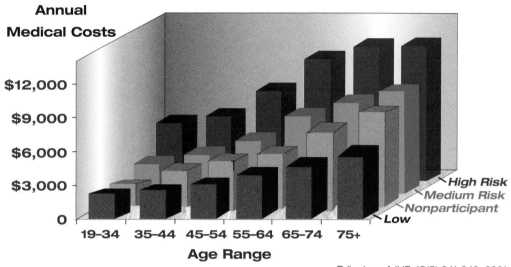

Edington. *AJHP*. 15(5):341-349, 2001.

This information sends a powerful message to companies (which receive aggregate data that is not specific to employees) and individuals (who receive personal, confidential health reports). This model has been replicated in dozens of companies, making it nearly impossible for anyone to argue that they can contain costs without initiating a health management effort.

We ask audiences the same two questions we raised in reference to the illness-wellness continuum, "Which bar do you want to be on?" and "Who is the leader to get you to that bar?" Everyone gets the picture.

Of course, not all diseases and costs can be prevented, but more of us will avoid them if we maintain a low-risk health status. Even people born with diabetes, for example, can be low risk if they watch what they eat, exercise, maintain a good body weight, and follow their diabetes treatment protocols.

Health Status as a Driver of Healthcare Costs

It is commonly accepted that as a group of people ages, the probability of disease increases, along with the cost of healthcare. In **Figure 7** (on page 46), the lower line demonstrates the typical association of medical costs with age: as age increases, medical costs increase. Some people propose "don't get old" as a solution, and it's too bad that is not a option. Yet, we certainly do not concur that we should accept the expectation that as we age, costs will invariably rise and health will deteriorate.

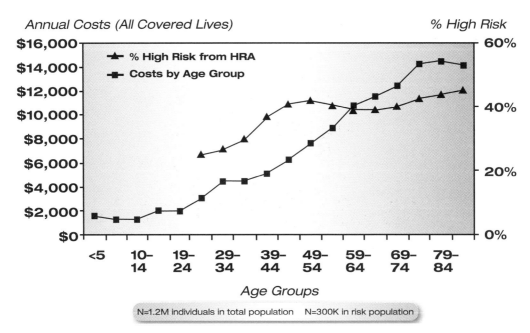

Figure 7. **Distribution: Age, Costs, & Risk Status**

University of Michigan Health Management Research Center

The upper line in Figure 7 shows the age-related increase in high risks in the population. That is, from age 25 to 55, the percent of the population at medium or high risk (three or more risks) increases from 20 percent to 40 percent (i.e., the age-related natural flow of risks in a population is from low risk to high risk). This graph suggests that the higher number of health risks may be of equal or perhaps even greater importance than aging as a cause of higher healthcare costs. Most individuals who have common chronic conditions (such as emphysema, heart disease, and diabetes) that lead to high sickness costs were not born with the risk factors that led to their illnesses; they accumulated them while living and working in American society. As people acquire more risk factors and health deteriorates, healthcare costs increase.

Summary

The charts in this chapter illustrate graphically the relationships between increasing health risk factors and increasing costs and suggest that disease and age are not the only factors behind increasing healthcare costs. Health risk factors often play a pivotal role. The evidence shows that the natural flow of health risks in the population is to high risk and the natural flow of costs in the population is to high cost.

> **It's clear that the cost of doing nothing is greater than**
> **the cost of doing something.**
> **The natural flow of risks is to high risk.**
> **The natural flow of costs is to high cost.**
> **Risks and costs increase with age.**

America has followed the sickness-oriented strategy for many decades, and that strategy has failed. One reason is that Americans have a natural tendency to develop more and more health risk factors over time; a second is that family, workplace, and community environments are often non-conducive to healthy and productive lifestyles. The cost of illness caused by poor health risk status far exceeds our capacity to pay. Together, the American health and economic situation has created a true crisis and unless America and Americans have the courage to change course the cost associated with illness will continue to increase. We must promote individual self-leaders who can reverse this trend.

Final Word

> **In society, we have a choice between focusing on disease (what's going**
> **wrong) or on the pursuit of vitality and health (what's going right).**
> **Seeking the solution of health solely through a focus on disease**
> **is like a dog or cat chasing its tail. It burns energy**
> **but brings about no meaningful results.**
> **It is time to stop this insanity.**

Chapter 5: *Health Management Is a Sustainable Strategy*

"We are at a point where it is impossible to do nothing."
—Helen Darling
President
National Business Group on Health

Developing a New Way of Thinking

When we talk with CEOs, company boards, and economic clubs, they understand the economic value of health status right away. What is the worth of a healthy and productive workforce? Would more companies survive and prosper if they fostered a healthy workplace? Would more companies come and fewer leave if a community were known for its healthy and productive population living and working with health integrated into the culture of the companies and community? Of course!

Changing the environments in which we live and work in order to reduce risk factors should be much easier than battling life-threatening illnesses and, perhaps even more importantly to everyone, it would avoid a tremendous amount of pain and suffering. Companies and individuals must understand that doing nothing is what allows the natural flow from low risk to high risk to disease to high cost. Therefore the ultimate solution, as demonstrated in **Figure 3** (on page 37), is to develop strategies to help the low-risk people stay low risk and to reverse the flow of individuals from low risk to high risk to disease. This is the essence of the new health status strategy.

Risks Associated with Disease

Diseases and costs are often driven by risk factors, and risk factors can be viewed individually or in combination with other risk factors. The data in **Figure 8** demonstrate an increased probability of diabetes in those with higher body weights (as indicated by BMI levels) as well as in those with a higher number of other risk factors. Although most of the publicity around the rising incidence of diabetes in this country attributes the problem to obesity, it's clear that regardless of body weight, additional health risks also are associated with a higher percentage of the population having diabetes.

If we want to reduce the number of adults who have Type 2 diabetes, we can focus either on reducing body weight, decreasing the number of other risk factors, or both. Studies over the past two decades demonstrate that weight loss alone is not likely to work.

Figure 8. Self-Reported Diabetes Associated with Levels of Body Mass Index

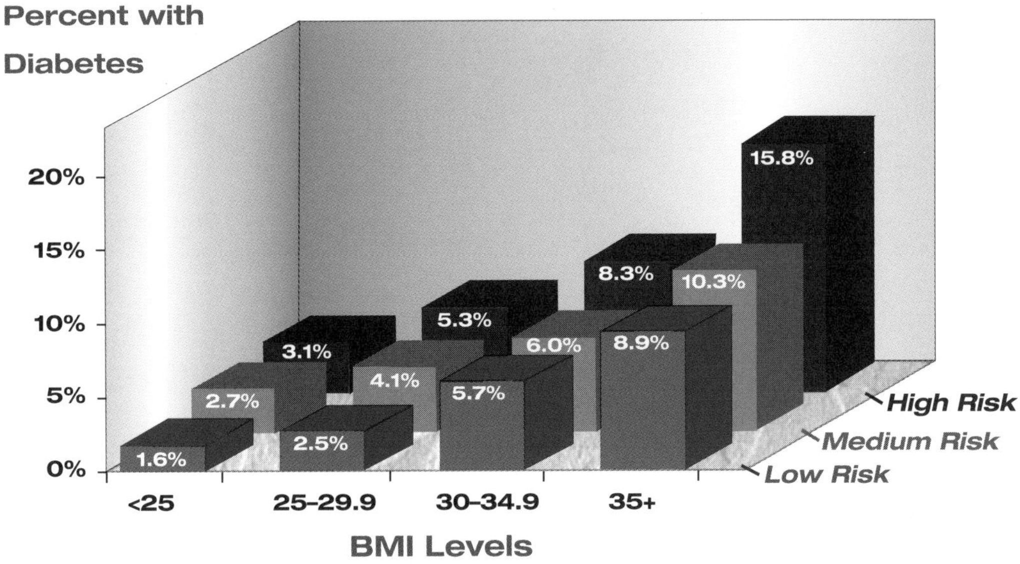

Musich, Lu, McDonald, Champagne, Edington. *AJHP.* 18(3):264-268, 2004.

The data in Figure 9 (on page 50) shows a similar picture. The percentage of people who have one or more of four major diseases (heart disease, diabetes, cancer, or emphysema/bronchitis) grows higher by age (which can't be controlled) or by an increased number of risk factors. Compared to the diabetes example above, only the number of risk factors can be modified.

In both of these examples, it is clear that a higher number of risk factors is associated with a higher probability of serious disease.

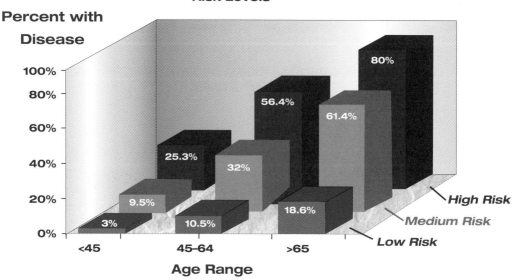

Figure 9. **Self-Reported Major Diseases Associated with Age and Risk Levels**

Musich, McDonald, Hirschland, Edington. *DM&HO.* 10(4):251-258, 2002.

Pay attention to people and their combined risks
in addition to individual risks or diseases.

Risks Associated with Costs

We published a series of studies and reports in the 1980s and 1990s around this simple premise: High numbers of risks are associated with high costs. Our goal was to observe the general pattern of the relationships. In nearly every case, individuals who were high risk in a single risk-factor category were high cost regardless of the outcome we were measuring. This held true for medical costs, pharmaceutical costs, days absent from work, days on disability, workers' compensation costs, or productivity.

However, in addition to the relative costs of high- and low-risk individuals for each risk factor, we found even more interesting and powerful data in the grouping of overall risk status. We classified people with zero to two health risks as low risk, people with three to four health risks as medium risk, and people with more than four risks as high risk. What we learned surprised us then and may surprise many readers now: Single, individual risk factors are not nearly as important as the combination of risks when it comes to predicting disease and high healthcare costs. These data were previously shown in Figure 6 (on page 45).

Risks Associated with Indicators of Productivity

Typically, we think of health risks and behaviors in terms of the way they impact medical and pharmacy costs, and that is certainly relevant. Now let's look at the ways these same risks impact other indicators that are crucial to the success of any company and its workers. We classify these as person-related productivity and put them into two major categories:

1. Time away from work (absenteeism)
2. Time lost while at work (presenteeism)

The data in Table 4 show that over a three-year period, manufacturing employees in the low-risk category–compared to their high-risk cohort–had a lower percent of people missing days of work due to absences, short- and long-term disability, workers' compensation, and total time away from work (61.3 percent compared to 81.7 percent). Likewise, Figure 10 (on page 52) shows that call center operators in the low-risk category had the least amount of lost time while at work (see the presenteeism component of the three bars in Figure 10). As we look at the absenteeism and presenteeism data, low-risk individuals are always the lowest cost and miss less work than the medium- or high-risk groups.

Table 4. Percentage of Employees with a Disability Claim Over a Three-Year Period*

HRA Participants 1998-2000 HRA	Low Risk 0-2 Risks (N=685)	Non- Participants (N=4,649)	Medium 3-4 Risks (N=520)	High Risk 5+ Risks (N=366)
WC Claims	25.4%	30.2%	30.2%	38.0%
STD Claims	23.4%	29.6%	30.8%	46.7%
Absence Record	49.9%	41.0%	63.1%	69.7%
Disability Claim	61.3%	64.4%	72.5%	81.7%

*Over three years 1998–2000

Wright, Beard, Edington. *JOEM.* 44(12):1126-1134, 2002.

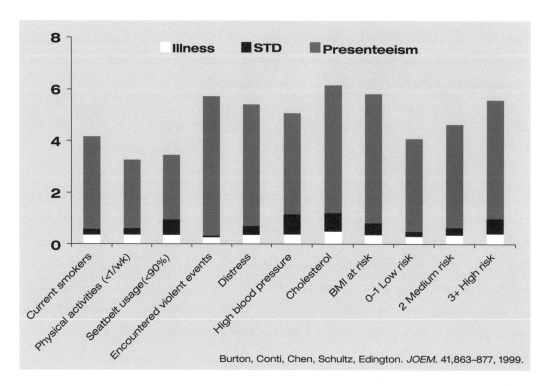

Figure 10. **Hours Lost Per Week**

Burton, Conti, Chen, Schultz, Edington. *JOEM*. 41,863–877, 1999.

Which Risks Travel with Other Risks

The several studies discussed in this section all confirm that it is not individual health risks or behaviors that result in the most costs but the accumulation and combinations of risk factors. It is also clear that high-risk status is most likely to cause high healthcare costs in the near future.

Intrigued by this finding, in the late 1990s and early 2000 we investigated which risk factors were most commonly associated with high-risk status. Not surprisingly, we discovered that some risks are more often associated with high-risk status than others. What did surprise us is that the risk most likely to travel with four other risks (thus making the individual overall high risk) is one's self-perception of health (see Table 5 on page 53). The least likely is body weight greater than a BMI of 27.5.

Clustering of Risks

The risk associations led us to explore the relationships: which risks travel together regardless of overall risk status? We identified four primary clusters: risk takers; low risk but with disease; biometric; and psychological. The clusters are illustrated in Table 6 (on page 54) The risk-takers are characterized by a high prevalence of smoking, not wearing seat belts, drinking higher levels of alcohol, etc.

They are somewhat younger and not prone to high healthcare costs within the next two to three years. Those individuals in the low-risk cluster have very few of the individual risks but a large number have chronic disease conditions. They also are unlikely to have high healthcare costs within the next two to three years.

Individuals who fall into the biometrics cluster, which includes combinations of high blood pressure, cholesterol, blood glucose, triglycerides and waist circumference, are those most likely to be at higher risk for heart disease or diabetes. This combination has now emerged in the medical literature as metabolic or cardiometabolic syndrome (CMS). Those who have three or more of the five risks are diagnosed as having CMS, which means they are close to getting diabetes or developing a heart condition. Individuals with one or two of the risks are considered pre-cardiometabolic syndrome. The flow diagram in Figure 11 (on page 55) is a good teaching tool for individuals and organizations to learn about the relationship of these risk factors with diabetes and heart disease. Notice that the arrows across the top are two directional, while the arrows going down are in one direction: Once your health is compromised to this extent, you cannot come back!

The questions are still: "Where do you want to be?" and "Where do you want your employees and their families to be?" and "Who is the leader to get you where you want to be?"

The individuals in the psychological cluster are more likely to have high body weight, be dissatisfied with their physical health, have relatively poor life satisfaction, be absent from work more

Table 5. Likelihood of Association with Other Risks

Population = 16,879 LifeSteps active screened participants	
Health Measure (among those at high risk)	**Percent in Overall High-Risk Category** (N-16,879)
Perceived health	68%
Life Satisfaction	52%
Stress	50%
Diastolic blood pressure	48%
Alcohol	45%
Systolic blood pressure	43%
Physical activity	41%
Safety belt	40%
Smoking	38%
Cholesterol	36%
HDL	34%
BMI	30%
Percentages show those at high risk for a particular health measure who have at least four other health risks.	

Braunstein, Yi, Hirschland, McDonald, Edington. *AJHB.* 25(4):407-417. 2001.

Table 6. **Cluster Analysis**

Health Measure	Cluster 1: Risk taking (N=6688)	Cluster 2: Low Risk (N=3164)	Cluster 3: Biometrics (N=3100)	Cluster 4: Psychological (N=3927)
Smoking	31%	0%	16%	27%
Alcohol	10%	0%	3%	5%
Physical activity	28%	0%	19%	26%
Safety belt usage	36%	0%	22%	31%
Body mass index	27%	25%	38%	27%
Systolic blood pressure	9%	0%	81%	23%
Diastolic blood pressure	5%	0%	61%	20%
Cholesterol	19%	19%	27%	22%
HDL cholesterol	34%	10%	33%	24%
Self-perceived health	13%	0%	9%	28%
Life satisfaction	4%	0%	2%	73%
Stress	9%	0%	2%	76%
Illness days	21%	0%	12%	26%
Overall Risks				
Low risk (0–2 risks)	50.2%	97.6%	26.5%	18.9%
Medium risk (3–4 risks)	35.7%	2.4%	48.9%	35.9%
High risk (5+ risks)	14.1%	0%	24.7%	45.2%
Average number of risks	2.8	0.6	3.6	4.4

Braunstein, Yi, Hirschland, McDonald, Edington. *AJHB.* 25(4):407-417, 2001.

often, and report high levels of stress. These individuals are likely headed toward mental health problems or even to depression.

The discovery of the cluster relationships points out the importance of the risk interactions and the potential consequences. For example, someone who is high risk for body weight and who is in the biometric cluster is likely going to be a high risk for diabetes while the person who is high risk for body weight but in the psychological cluster could be possibly headed toward a mental health issue. Therefore, cluster-specific approaches to coaching these individuals would be appropriate.

Prioritization of Risks

We have demonstrated that higher numbers of risks are associated with higher healthcare costs and with lower productivity. Also, risks tend to travel together and form definable clusters. The natural question is then, "Can the risks be prioritized in order to identify the most critical risk leading to higher cost or disease?"

Figure 11. Relationship of Biometric Cluster to Diabetes and Heart Disease

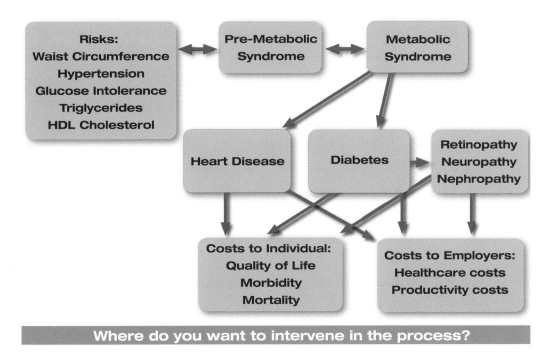

Where do you want to intervene in the process?

There are several stratification methods that could be used, such as:

1. Listing all the individual risks for each person

2. Grouping the individuals by the total number of risks

3. Using a prioritization engine to rank order the risks in terms of their impact on costs or disease within the next two to three years.

Option one is stratification without prioritization. Option two is to prioritize individuals into low-, medium-, and high-risk status. This option prioritizes the highest overall risk individuals without ranking the individual risks.

Option three requires a much more sophisticated set of algorithms in order to prioritize the risks according to their impact on future costs or disease for each individual. This stratification reveals a set of dangerous risk combinations which lead to higher costs. The distribution of the risks within these combinations allows us to prioritize the risks for each individual. The overall probability of future high cost can be calculated and the individual's rank order within the population from most likely to least likely to be high cost over the next two to three years.

When individuals are ranked and predicted to be high cost, the projection is correct between 70 percent and 83 percent of the time. Among persons predicted to be low cost, the model shows approximately a 10 percent error rate; that is, 10 percent of those expected to be low-cost turn out to be high-cost. The specific science behind option three is the intellectual property of the University of Michigan and has been exclusively licensed to CIGNA. However, it exemplifies one of the ways that the valuable HRA data can be put to use, and we challenge others to move in this more scientific direction. We need other methods to challenge all of us to get as far in front of pain and suffering and high cost as possible. We do not need another generation of people living while waiting for sickness.

Options one and two are commonly used in the health management field. We also developed option two, which has been widely published in the literature, and it is the stratification used in many of the existing and more advanced HRA instruments. Option two is used to calculate excess costs due to excess risks, as explained in the next paragraph.

Excess Costs Are Associated with Excess Risks in Individuals

High-risk status, most often caused by an accumulation of risks, gives way to the concept that excess risks cause higher costs. When we compare the costs of medium- and high-risk individuals to those of low-risk individuals, a cost differential can be identified as "excess costs due to excess risks." In a series of studies in the 1990s, we found this relationship to be true for all of the cost outcomes we measured. That is, additional risks are associated with higher costs for medical care, pharmacy,

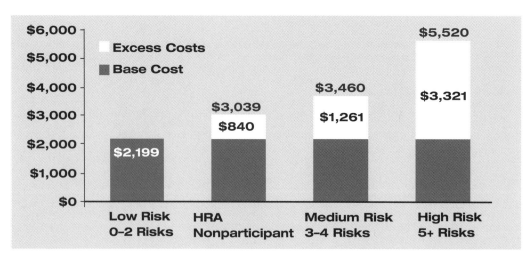

Figure 12. **Excess Medical Costs Due to Excess Risks**

Edington. *AJHP*. 15(5):341-349, 2001.

days absent from work, disability and workers' compensation claims, and overall productivity while at work. When populations are separated into categories of risk status, the low-risk status group forms the baseline, with each higher-risk status group showing excess costs due to excess risk factors. Figure 12 gives an example of this concept using medical and pharmacy costs only.

Working with our Corporate Consortium companies over more than 25 years enabled us to collect enough long-term data to examine trends in new ways. In one study of six corporations, we found that the companies were paying 15 to 31 percent higher healthcare costs due to excess risks. As we continued to study risk factors within groups of employees, it became clear that each risk factor added costs. A comprehensive study of about 100,000 General Motors employees found that individuals who had excess risk factors had excess healthcare costs, with or without an existing disease. For those who did have an existing disease, more risk factors meant even more added costs. For example, high-risk people with diabetes had 19 percent higher healthcare costs than diabetics who did not have excess risks.

"The data illustrating the healthcare costs of people who are high risk vs. those who are low risk tells the whole story. We are the payers on this, and our costs are going to go through the roof if we don't get control of those risk factors or keep people healthy."

—*J. Brent Pawlecki, MD*
Corporate Medical Director
Pitney Bowes, Inc.

Using Excess Costs to Get to the Total Value of Health Risk to a Company

We have studied excess costs in each of our Corporate Consortium companies. One of several studies at Steelcase showed that excess risks accounted for 36 percent of costs when we totaled the costs for medical, pharmacy, absence, disability, and workers' compensation (see Table 7 on page 58). This type of calculation begins to reveal what could be saved if a company launches an effective strategy to create a culture of health. And it's only the beginning. Consider the value of measures that weren't included in that study, including increased productivity while at work, better recruitment and retention outcomes, and cost savings from having healthy spouses and dependents.

Understanding that excess risks account for increased costs is as important to individuals as it is for businesses. We can determine which individuals, based on their health risk status, are heading

Table 7. Association of Risk Levels with Corporate Cost Measures

Outcome Measure	Low Risk	Medium Risk	High Risk	Excess Cost Percentage
Short-term Disability	$ 120	$ 216	$ 333	41%
Workers' Compensation	$ 228	$ 244	$ 496	24%
Absence	$ 245	$ 341	$ 527	29%
Medical & Pharmacy	$1,158	$1,487	$3,696	38%
Total	$1,751	$2,288	$5,052	36%

Wright, Beard, Edington. *JOEM*. 44(12):1126-1134, 2002.

for high-cost episodes of healthcare and, more importantly, avoidable pain and suffering. (This determination requires the HMRC's more sophisticated analytics, which are not described in this book.)

So, knowing that high-risk individuals are high-cost individuals, and excess risks lead to excess costs, the next question is, "If I change my risk in either direction, will my costs follow in the same direction?" That is, "If I reduce my risks, will I lower my costs?"

What's important about this "excess costs due to excess risks" concept is that it means much of what individuals and companies spend on healthcare, or sickness care, is excess relative to a baseline of zero to two risks. The natural extension of this concept would be to find a way to move everyone to low-risk status. The excess dollars would not have to be spent if no one in the population had excess risks. It may be difficult to imagine that we could move everyone in the population to low-risk status and keep them there, but we believe it's possible. In the third section, we'll provide a total strategy for making this happen.

Changes in healthcare costs follow changes
in health risk in the same direction.
As the number of risks goes up, costs go up.
As the number of risks goes down, costs go down.

Total Value of Health

The primary health outcome measures that concern companies the most are medical (inpatient and outpatient) and pharmaceutical costs. In 2003, the HMRC published the first of many papers establishing the total value of health to an organization. The idea that promoting and maintaining a healthy population produces an economic return on investment was, and still is, a revelation in many corporate circles. The total sum of the costs in Figure 13 includes those costs for medical and pharmacy; time away from work (absence, short- and long-term disability, and workers' compensation); and presenteeism (time lost while at work because health risks or disease impacts one's ability to complete work-related tasks). Other factors such as how health status impacts monetary costs related to recruitment, retention, and morale are not estimated.

At General Motors, Joel Bender MD, PhD, Corporate Medical Director, states that "We are looking at the costs of sub-optimum health in a number of areas. For example, absence from work due to claimed disability is an important area for us. On too many workdays, we have more than one in twenty hourly workers absent. Obviously, disability plan design and work rules can be a major driver. However, we want to make sure that we are reasonably supporting our employees' healthy choices and habits that might avoid or minimize these absences. Our actions include encouraging employees

Figure 13. Relative Costs of the Total Value of Health

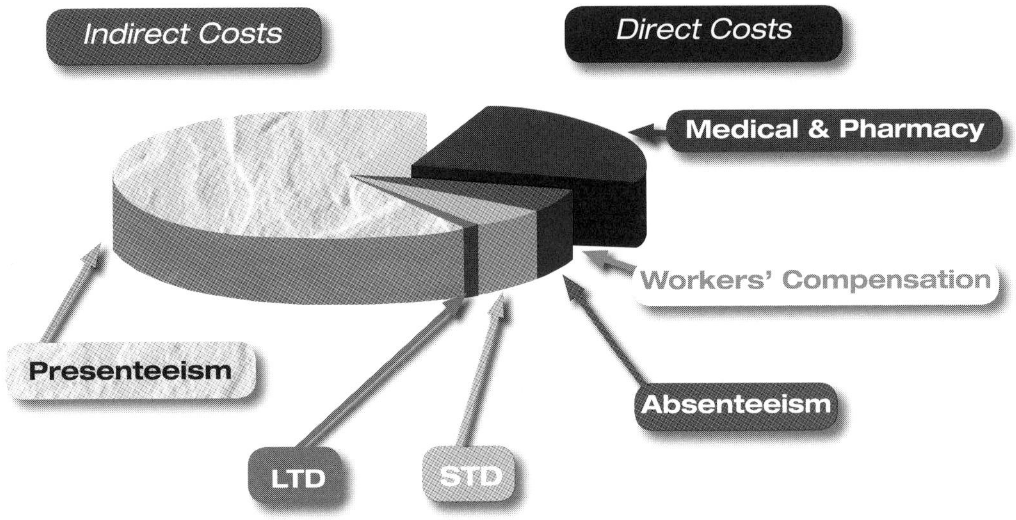

Edington, Burton. A Practical Approach to Occupational and Environmental Medicine (McCunny). 140-152. 2003.

to eat healthy foods in moderate quantities, to eliminate or reduce tobacco use, to exercise frequently but moderately, and to take advantage of excellent preventive health services. When employees are unfortunately sick or injured, whether occurring at work, play, or home, we support them to get healthy again and to return to work as soon as is it is safe to do so. An integrated health care approach that involves coaches that support compliance and health improvement for specific disorders such as asthma, diabetes, and congestive heart failure has proven to be very effective.

Economic Costs to Individuals and Organizations

The major question that has driven the development of this new health management strategy is:

"How does health status, and more importantly change in health status, impact economic and human costs to individuals and organizations?"

Now that we have described the impact of risks on costs, the next thing organizations and individuals want to know is: "How far upstream do I want to begin my investment?"

"The critical measure of success is health status. The evidence is conclusive that costs follow risks, so the key data to measure for companies of all sizes is the health of their population. If the trend indicates an improvement in overall health risks, the benefits will follow in terms of lower healthcare costs and improved productivity measures."

—Stephen Cherniak
Wellness Director
Strategic Benefit Solutions

For years, companies intuitively invested in the medium- and high-risk people, trying to change their unhealthy behaviors and thus lower healthcare costs. Now, we know there is a much better strategy, as Figure 3 (on page 37) indicates. The only logical answer to where to begin, based on our research, is to increase our investment in the low-risk category.

The natural flow of risks and costs also explains why the do-nothing strategy will only lead to greater amounts of disease and higher costs. We must create strategies to maintain low-risk populations within our homes, businesses, and communities

To an individual, the consequences of high-risk health status and disease are obvious: low energy and vitality, a high amount of pain and suffering, stress, reduced quality of life, limited mobility and independence, and financial instability. To an organization, the consequences of high-risk health status and disease can be calculated by looking at the even broader value of an employee's health. When an employee is sick, an employer who is providing health insurance pays much more than medical and drug bills alone. The cost of high-risk status and disease includes medical and pharmaceutical costs, days absent from work, short- and long-term disability costs, workers' compensation, and reduced productivity while at work. Also, factor in disruption to the normal flow of productivity within the employee's work group and possibly the whole company. It is relatively obvious to see the value of supporting and maintaining individuals at low risk and helping the healthy people stay healthy.

"On one hand, it IS rocket science to analyze current disease and health risks to project the future with great certainty. On the other hand, the clear results are not; maintain or reduce health risks and cost reductions will follow."

Neal Sofian
Director, Behavior Health Interventions
Resolution Health, Inc.

Final Word

Health management is a health strategy, but equally important, health management is a business and economic strategy.

Chapter 6: *It Works: Getting Better by Not Getting Worse*

"Not to go back is somewhat to advance, and men must walk, at least, before they dance."
—Alexander Pope

This chapter completes the brief review of our first 30 years of work, summarized by the statement that "when risk status changes or when participation in health promotion activities changes, costs follow in the same direction." Even when risk status stays the same rather than getting worse, costs remain constant or even are reduced. The data also show that just getting people engaged in activities results in lower increases in all of the economic outcome measures.

Thus, we discovered another summary statement, "…getting better by not getting worse." For the purposes of this book, we selected only a limited number of our studies to demonstrate the critical relationships for building the business case for health management programs. All of our studies and the studies of others can be found in our research companion book: *Cost-Benefit of Health Management Programs 1979 to 2009.*

Benefits for Individuals and Organizations

Americans demand too little from the current healthcare system when they merely ask, "Cure me when I get sick." Americans should expect more: "I want a full life of vitality and energy and to be relatively free from pain and suffering." Americans can achieve high health status, along with very substantial economic benefits, such as fewer lost wages, fewer expensive medical bills, more quality time with their families, and a longer life expectancy. Of course, reducing the pain and suffering of family members is reason enough to support an individual's quest for better health.

"Proving that this is a good investment for business is going to help to prove that it's a good social invest-ment as well. This kind of thinking will ultimately lead us to save money, but it will also improve people's capacity to lead meaningful lives."

—*Sean Sullivan*
President and CEO
Institute of Health and Productivity Management

Wellness Score Is an Indicator of Medical and Pharmacy Costs

There are many health risk appraisals on the market. The best versions have a comprehensive score beyond a flat calculation of risks. The HRA developed by the University of Michigan Health Management Research Center is no exception. Our wellness score is calculated using three primary components:

1. **Number of high-risk areas**
2. **Percent of recommended preventive services completed**
3. **A composite score from calculations based the interactions of the risks**

The details of the University of Michigan HRA Wellness Score have been referenced in many peer-reviewed papers. The score-cost data in Figure 14 (on page 64) shows the relatively linear inverse relationship between the wellness scores and medical and pharmacy costs: the higher the well-ness score, the lower the healthcare costs.

Change in Costs Follow Change in Wellness Score

From the mid-1970s, when HRA's first came into use, through the mid 2000s, health pro-motion companies attempted to improve the health of their clients entirely through risk reduction. Although we know that a change in risk will result in a change in cost, the strategy of focusing on risk reduction alone is flawed. This is because costs follow risks in both directions. You may succeed in reducing one high-risk behavior while overlooking another area where risk is moving from low to high. A common example is the person who quits smoking but gains weight, and with that develops high blood pressure. If one risk goes down as others increase, the result is a near zero and perhaps a negative net change. The flow chart in Figure 15 (on page 65) illustrates how changes in the well-

Figure 14. **Relationship Between Annual Medical and Pharmacy Costs and Wellness Score**

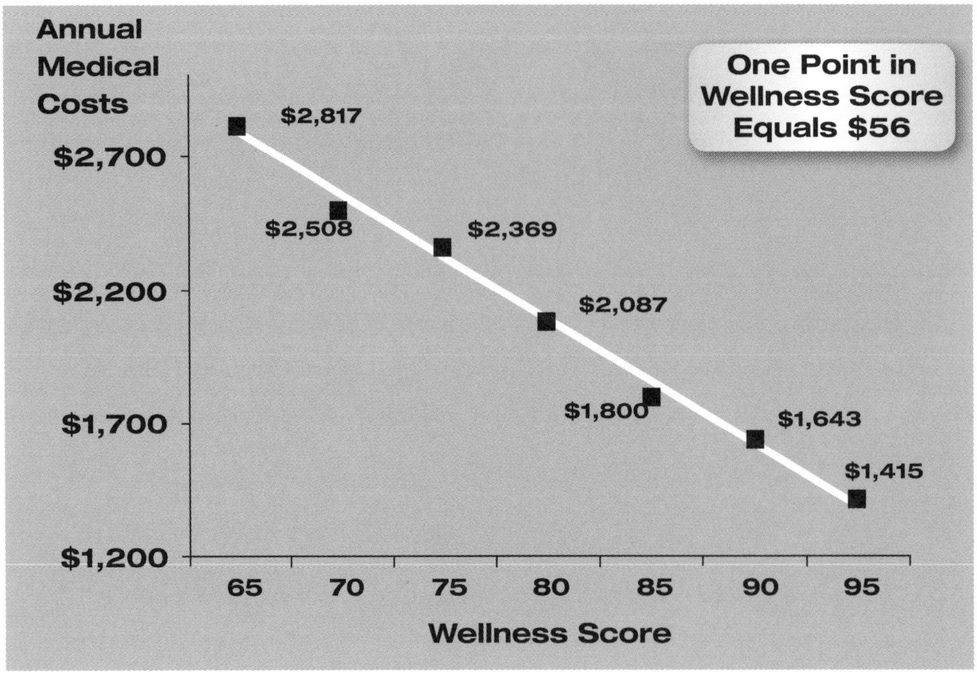

Yen, McDonald, Hirschland, Edington. JOEM. 45(10):1049-1057, 2003.

ness score are reflected in changes in medical and pharmacy costs year after year. That is, the higher the wellness score (100 is excellent, and 50 is poor), the lower the costs; the lower the wellness score, the higher the costs. In every case, as wellness scores change from one year to the next, costs change in the opposite direction.

Change in Costs Follow Change in Risks

Even over short periods of time, when risks change, costs change in the same direction. However, when the number of risks increase the costs increase faster than they decrease when risks decrease. For illustrative purposes we have shown only the changes in medical/drug costs in Figure 16. The interesting thing is that the pattern seems to be the same regardless of which risk changes. This just reinforces our belief that it is not the specific risks but the patterns of the risks that drive costs.

Figure 15. Wellness Score and Costs over 3 Years

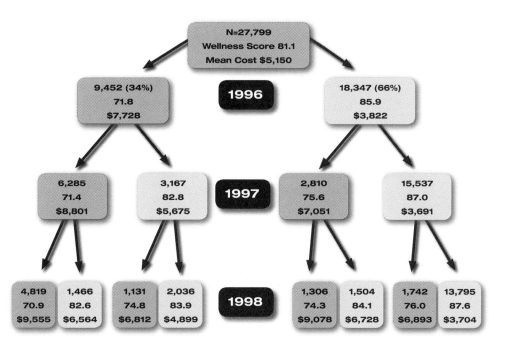

Figure 16. Change in Costs Follow Change in Risks

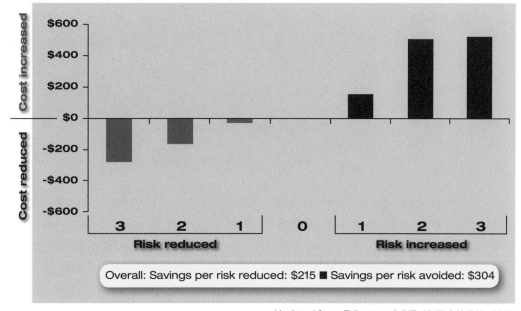

Updated from Edington, *AJHP*. 15(5):341-349, 2001.

Change in Costs Follows Participation

The HMRC has tracked the effectiveness of participating in health promotion programs in a number of longitudinal studies. Figures 17 and 18 show the results of following two groups of employees in two manufacturing companies. In one company, we followed medical/drug costs of more than 3,000 employees for ten years. Our findings show that those who completed an HRA at least twice over the ten years had an annual increase in costs of 4.2 percent, while those who never took the HRA or took it just once showed annual increases of 12.6 percent.

Figure 17. **Annual Cost Increase Associated with Program Involvement from 1985 to 1995**

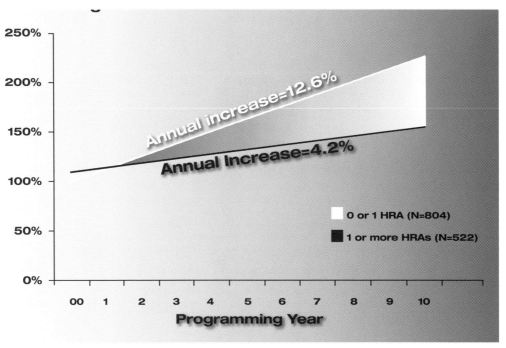

University of Michigan Health Management Research Center

Similarly, we looked at employees at two manufacturing plants who took advantage of their companies' wellness programs. The average annual increase in absent days over the five years of the study was 2.4 percent for the participating employees compared to 3.6 percent for the nonparticipation employees. The savings related to participation in wellness programs were calculated to exceed $300,000 per plant over those five years plus associated healthcare costs along with the higher morale that is typically associated with engagement in health management programs.

Figure 18. Yearly Average Disability Absence Days by Participation

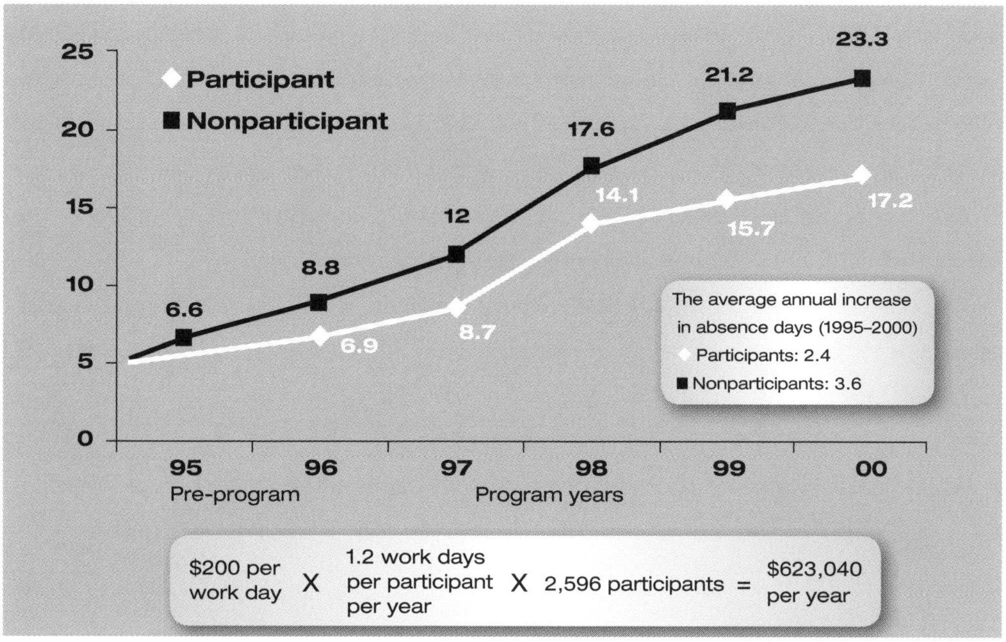

◆ **Participant**
■ **Nonparticipant**

23.3
21.2
17.6
17.2
15.7
14.1
12
8.8
8.7
6.9
6.6

The average annual increase
in absence days (1995–2000)
◆ Participants: 2.4
■ Nonparticipants: 3.6

25
20
15
10
5
0

95   96   97   98   99   00
Pre-program   Program years

| $200 per work day | X | 1.2 work days per participant per year | X | 2,596 participants | = | $623,040 per year |

Schultz, Musich, McDonald, Hirschland, Edington. *JOEM.* 44(8):776-780, 2002.

Figure 19. The Influence of Health Status on Total Cost

(A Human Capital Approach)

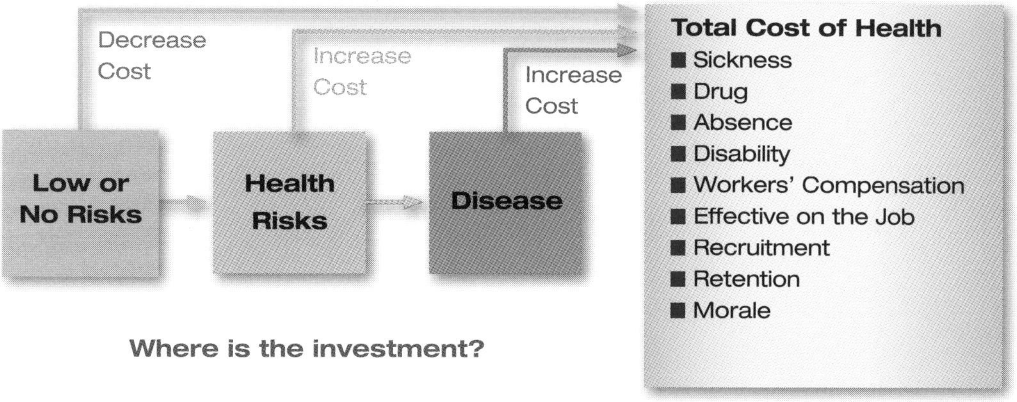

Decrease
Cost

Increase
Cost

Increase
Cost

**Low or
No Risks**   →   **Health
Risks**   →   **Disease**

Total Cost of Health
■ Sickness
■ Drug
■ Absence
■ Disability
■ Workers' Compensation
■ Effective on the Job
■ Recruitment
■ Retention
■ Morale

Where is the investment?

University of Michigan Health Management Research Center

The Case for Organizations

The total cost of healthcare to the individual and to the organization is determined by the flow of people from low risk to high risk. High risk is a very short distance from disease and high cost (see Figure 19 on page 67). Each company has the opportunity to devise the most effective strategy to maintain the health and productivity of the workplace and workforce. The current situation of waiting for employees to get sick is untenable. Healthcare will go through a transformation when effective strategies are in place for helping individuals further upstream, preferably while health is good and before they enter into the high-risk to disease to high-cost cycle.

The objective is to create an enhanced environment in which the workplace and workforce become part of a health-promoting culture that helps the healthy people stay healthy. Anyone in business understands that:

It is easier to keep a good customer than to try to find a new one.
In this case, the low-risk individuals are the good customers.

Just Don't Get Worse

One of our most enlightening and interesting findings, and the rationale for our "don't get worse" theme, is that individuals whose health improves or remains stable get to what we call zero trend. This means that their healthcare cost increases do not exceed the corresponding rise in the average price of consumer goods and services purchased by households. The data in Figure 20 (on page 69) show that when individuals change in a positive direction or "don't get worse," their costs (medical and pharmacy) stay the same or drop lower. When they change in a "get worse" direction, their costs go up. Employees who "don't get worse" approach zero trend in year-to-year costs.

"We have a goal to drive the trend of healthcare cost increases to zero. We are going to do it by ensuring that we understand the personal health and vitality of every employee as well as the health and vitality of organizations."

—*Catherine Rieger*
Senior Director, Product Development Specialist
CIGNA Corp.

Figure 20. Improved Employees Approach Zero Trend in Cost

Medical and Drug Cost (Paid)*

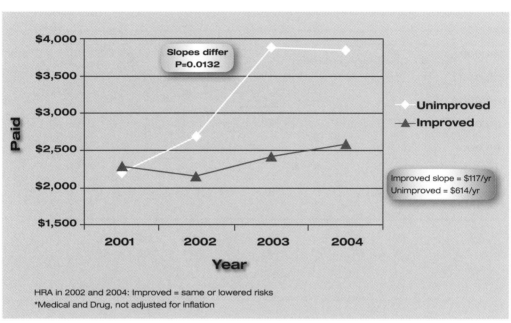

HRA in 2002 and 2004: Improved = same or lowered risks
*Medical and Drug, not adjusted for inflation

University of Michigan Health Management Research Center

Zero Trend

Another way to view this finding is illustrated by Figure 21 (on page 70), reproduced from Figure 7 (on page 46). The percent of the population at low risk is shown on the top curve. If you assume that this group of people does not get worse, the horizontal arrow represents their status over the next several years. It is obvious that **by not getting worse one is actually getting better**. And on the cost curve (lower line), we have projected the resulting **zero trend**.

The arrows in Figure 21 indicate that when the population consciously decides to "not get worse," in reality they are getting better compared to where they would have been if they continue to do nothing. When people do not get worse in terms of their health status, they approach zero trend in terms of healthcare costs.

Figure 21. To Not Get Worse Approaches Zero Trend
Distribution: Age, Costs, and Risk Status

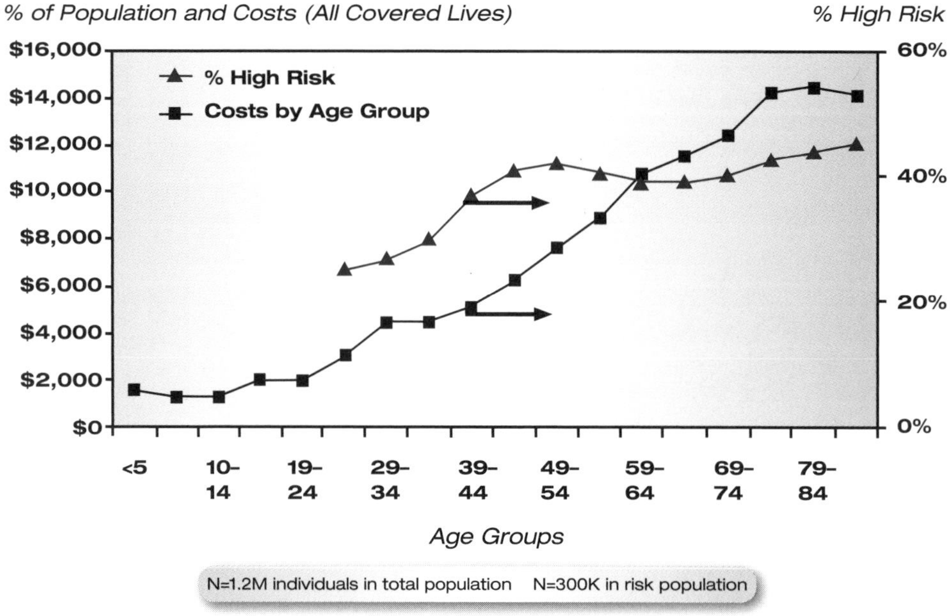

% of Population and Costs (All Covered Lives)   % High Risk

N=1.2M individuals in total population   N=300K in risk population

University of Michigan Health Management Research Center

Summary to This Section

Helping companies recognize that they can create economic value by investing in healthy and productive people has been at the core of the HMRC's work since its inception. Our studies show that if individuals and corporations as well as communities, states, and the nation all work together, we can turn the tide of declining health status and overwhelming healthcare and productivity costs. The key is to manage health risk factors before disease strikes.

Excess costs are related to excess risks.

Costs follow engagement and risks.

Controlling risks leads to zero trend.

Figure 22. **Health Management Research Center**

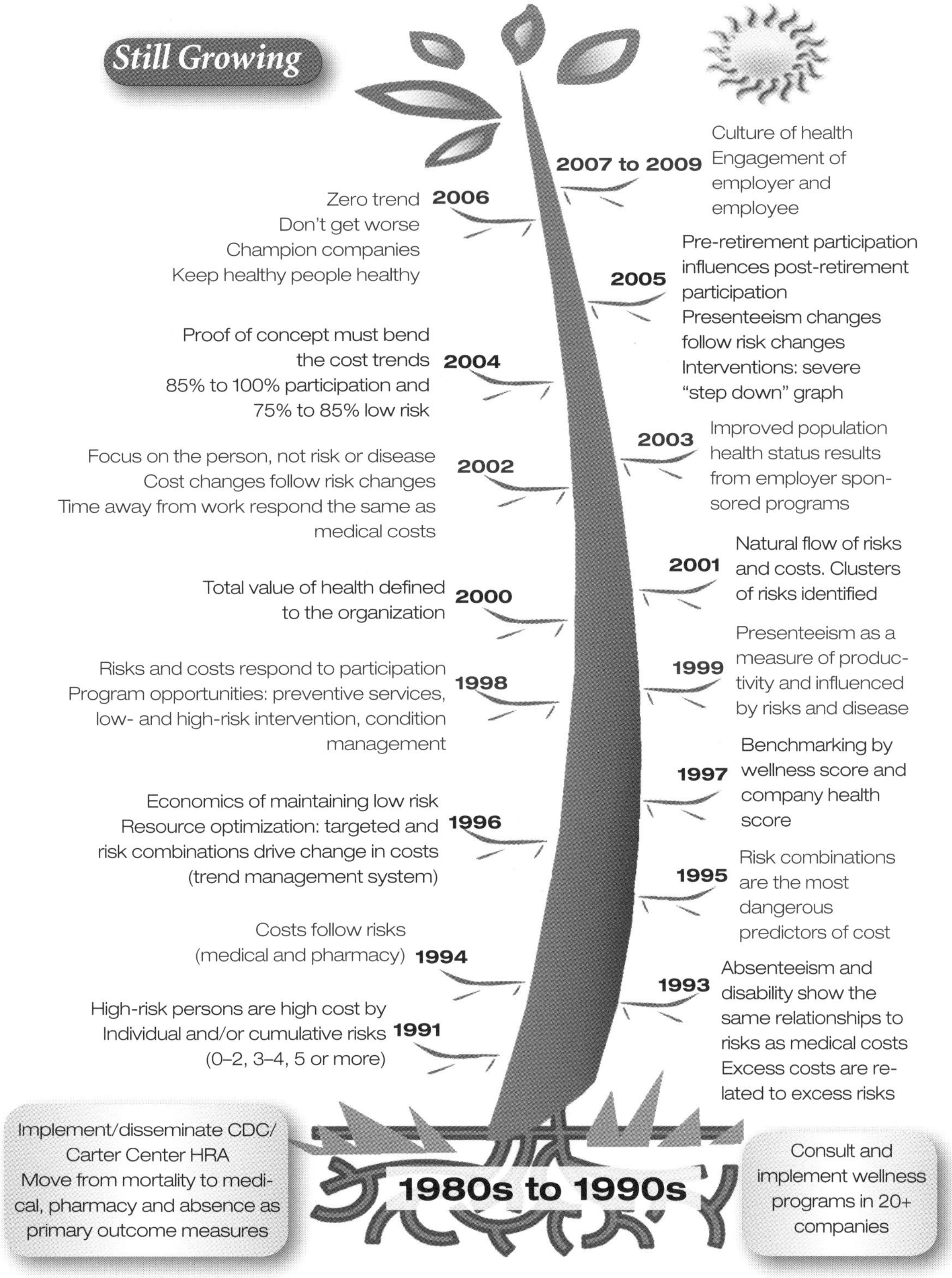

Still Growing

2007 to 2009
Culture of health
Engagement of
employer and
employee

Zero trend **2006**
Don't get worse
Champion companies
Keep healthy people healthy

2005
Pre-retirement participation
influences post-retirement
participation
Presenteeism changes
follow risk changes
Interventions: severe
"step down" graph

Proof of concept must bend
the cost trends **2004**
85% to 100% participation and
75% to 85% low risk

2003
Improved population
health status results
from employer spon-
sored programs

Focus on the person, not risk or disease **2002**
Cost changes follow risk changes
Time away from work respond the same as
medical costs

2001
Natural flow of risks
and costs. Clusters
of risks identified

Total value of health defined **2000**
to the organization

1999
Presenteeism as a
measure of produc-
tivity and influenced
by risks and disease

Risks and costs respond to participation
Program opportunities: preventive services, **1998**
low- and high-risk intervention, condition
management

1997
Benchmarking by
wellness score and
company health
score

Economics of maintaining low risk
Resource optimization: targeted and **1996**
risk combinations drive change in costs
(trend management system)

1995
Risk combinations
are the most
dangerous
predictors of cost

Costs follow risks
(medical and pharmacy) **1994**

1993
Absenteeism and
disability show the
same relationships to
risks as medical costs
Excess costs are re-
lated to excess risks

High-risk persons are high cost by
Individual and/or cumulative risks **1991**
(0–2, 3–4, 5 or more)

1980s to 1990s

Implement/disseminate CDC/
Carter Center HRA
Move from mortality to medical, pharmacy and absence as
primary outcome measures

Consult and
implement wellness
programs in 20+
companies

The "limbs on the tree" in Figure 22 (on page 71) illustrate the HMRC research findings over the decades of the 1980s, 1990s, and 2000s. Our work has been systematic and focused on health as an economic outcome for individuals and corporations. Similar to growing any plant or tree, one has to "till the soil," which we did for nearly a decade to establish the relationship between health risks and behaviors with higher medical and productivity costs; some of these results show up on the lower branches of the tree. The next series of studies was related to finding out that when risks change, costs change in the same direction. During this time we also discovered the cluster stratification technique. Our most advanced and sophisticated algorithms are in the Trend Management System, which allows us to identify for each individual the most important risk that, once addressed, will produce the most cost savings over the next two to three years. Finally, our predictive modeling in our Medical Economics Report produces results to model population results according to one of four intensities (engagement levels will be discussed in Chapter 7) of program intervention.

Final Word

We have established the failures of the wait for sickness strategy.

We have documented the promises of the health management strategy.

We have examined the economics of a new way to do health management.

We have therefore established the evidence to move toward the solution.

It is time to answer the question,

"How do we create the culture and programs that will produce the benefits?"

And now that we all get it, it's the perfect time to act!

The Solution: *Integrating Health Status into the Company Culture*

Five Fundamental Pillars to Support a Culture of Health

"Intellectuals solve problems, geniuses prevent them."
—*Albert Einstein*

Guidelines for Reading This Section

Based upon our research findings, we describe the five fundamental pillars of an evidence-based strategy designed to integrate health status into the culture of the workplace. The objective is to facilitate high-level health status for all employees, economically benefiting both individuals and their companies. Within each pillar, we present four evidence-based levels of program engagement for organizations to use in deciding to select their investment strategy and to measure their results.

It is unlikely that any company would be in a position to address each of the five fundamental pillars and achieve champion company engagement level within the first or second year. However, efforts within each of the five pillars are absolutely necessary—even within the first year—with the goal of achieving champion company status within three years. This section does not aim to provide a tool kit of resources, but to share the process for the leaders of any size company to implement within their own culture.

Chapter 7: *Integrating Health Status into the Culture*

The Five Fundamental Pillars and Company Engagement Levels

"Having a culture of health at Pitney Bowes has been my passion throughout my 18 years as a senior leader at the company. As an employer, we can have a major impact on the health and well-being of our employees, and we have systematically acted to achieve that goal since 1990. Investment in health delivery is consistent with a long-term view of maximizing return on human capital. However, prioritizing health-related investments is key."

—Michael J. Critelli
CEO and Chairman
Pitney Bowes, Inc.

Companies Need a Sustainable Solution

American corporations are coming to a full understanding that success in this increasingly competitive and economically challenged world depends on a healthy and productive workplace and workforce. And the employees themselves are in the early stages of realizing that they can improve their lives and the lives of their family members by becoming self-leaders, taking charge of their own health status.

Yet, whatever we do has to be done quickly, because the current healthcare strategy is unsustainable. The time is now, and the systems are in place for regaining our vitality and our competitive advantage. We need the entire population on board, thinking at a higher level about the total value of health! Walter Talamonti, Medical Director of Clinical Operations at Ford Motor Company, emphasizes this same point. "We cannot continue to pay double-digit increases in healthcare, so we have to look at what will ultimately reduce the costs. You can't just keep cutting what you offer. You have to do something different. One of the company's top strategies for controlling those costs in the next several years is to roll out its wellness program. The goal is to create a culture of health within the company."

George Pfeiffer, President and CEO of The WorkCare Group, Inc., has been in this field for more than 35 years and he has seen the evidence that, "Today, through health and productivity management we are able to measure objectively that which, as practitioners, we knew intuitively 35 years ago—healthy employees cost less and are more productive. Yet, in spite of this wealth of data, comprehensive employee health management programs are almost exclusive to large employers. To truly align the concept of a culture of health within the employer space, small- and medium-size employers need to be engaged, which requires revised program models and service delivery." We would agree with him that the percentage of larger companies having health management programs is greater than that of the small- and medium-size companies. However, based on our criteria, most programs, regardless of size, are in what we will call level 1—minimal and not a serious business strategy to make it effective and sustainable. The problem may be rooted within some of the vendor health enhancement companies as they continue to sell only those products they currently market rather than developing creative products that are needed to meet the specific needs of their client companies.

Effective strategic leadership in the organization must come from the top. Only engagement and commitment at this level can transform the vision into reality. Eventually, communities and states will realize the economic and social value of a healthy and productive citizenry and appreciate the total value of this effort.

What It Takes to Succeed

Our goal is to convince organizations to make health an integral part of the corporate culture. Working with our Corporate Consortium and other companies over three decades, we've learned what it takes to succeed. The health management strategies must be driven by three levels: senior leadership, operations leadership, and the employees practicing self-leadership. Equally important are reward and quality assurance systems that measure and ensure sustainable success. These three populations and two key strategies combine to form the five fundamental pillars of success.

The following is paraphrased from a philosophy we encountered while conducting a session for the medical directors of a large manufacturing company. It captures the essence of what this book is about: connecting people to products and to mission.

Our mission is to create shareholder value. We create shareholder value because we have innovative, creative, and quality products and services. We have innovative, creative, and quality products and services because we have healthy and productive people.

A Culture That Engages the Total Population

Finding the right solution for the right person at the right time is absolutely necessary in order to gain widespread commitment. Employers need to offer benefit coverage and other services that meet the individual needs of their entire populations. The full slate begins with services for enabling people to "not get worse" and then helping them take steps to improve their current health status, regardless of where they fall on one of the three lines in Figure 23. These services range from resources for helping healthy people stay healthy, to helping those who are sick get through their acute crisis, to helping those coping with chronic disease or illness either obtain full recovery or maintain their best possible health status. The most progressive corporations engage partners (not vendors) to offer programs for each one of these groups.

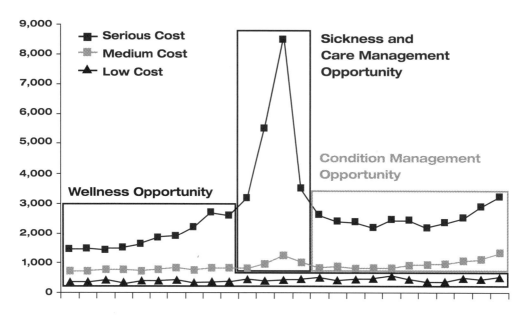

Figure 23. Provide Benefits to Cover All Employees
Medical and Drug Costs Only

Musich, Schultz, Burton, Edington. *DM&HO.* 12(5):299–326, 2004.

"Like most corporations, Xerox is too familiar with the specter of ever increasing healthcare costs. But companies can't solve the problem alone. Our healthcare business strategy today—evolved from our long history of supporting a healthy workforce and workplace—is built on further strengthening the employee value proposition and specifically, investing in tools that help guide employees to actively manage their health. "

—*Anne M. Mulcahy*
CEO and Chairman
Xerox Corporation

It is necessary to bring together all available resources and provide assistance that leads each person to the right resource at the right time. For example, Florida Power & Light offers a "wheel" of resources covering many, but not necessarily all, of the programs and services organizations can make available to their populations (see Figure 24). Even smaller companies can combine their own

Figure 24. **Create an Integrated and Sustainable Approach**

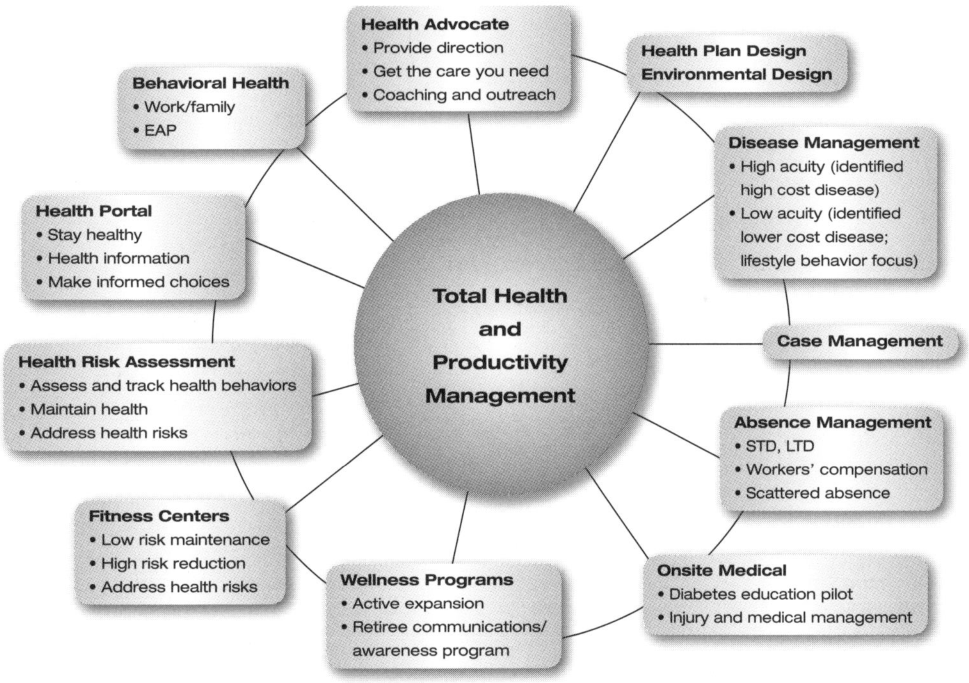

Long Term Strategy—Short Term Solutions

resources with those found in the community. As the diagram demonstrates, all available resources have to be integrated and focused on the total environment if health is to be integrated into the culture. The program must be accessible to all employees and their family members, and then it has to be sustainable.

"If American employers solve some of these productivity matters, our employees are going to be healthier, much more productive, and we'll be able to compete worldwide very effectively."

—*Pete Petit*

Former Chairman and CEO

Matria Healthcare

Addressing the Supportive Environment

We know that if individuals are to make a sustainable behavior change, they must be in an environment that supports that change. If someone changes a behavior and then returns to the same unhealthy environment that caused or aggravated the behavior, the chances are pretty good that they will return to their original behavior. Despite all of the psychological evidence that this is true, many

Figure 25. **Health Management in the Workplace**

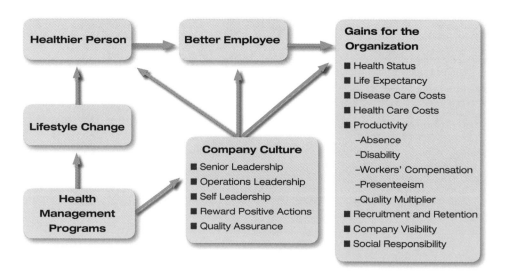

behavior change professionals persist in focusing only on the person and the problem, and overlook the place where the problem is happening.

Effective and sustainable behavior change efforts must encompass the overall culture of the workplace. Figure 25 (on page 78) shows how this integration forms the centerpiece of a health management program in a champion company. Five fundamental pillars, as we describe next, support the health management activity.

Five Fundamental Pillars

Support a Successful Health Management Strategy

This health management strategy incorporates all of our research and everything we've talked about in this book. It can enable companies and their total population to maximize the potential of their optimal health. The 30 years of scientific findings referenced in the previous sections led us to these evidence-based recommendations. The fundamental idea is to integrate the health management strategy into the environment and culture of an organization. The strategy is built on the five pillars of success described in Table 8.

Table 8. The Five Fundamental Pillars

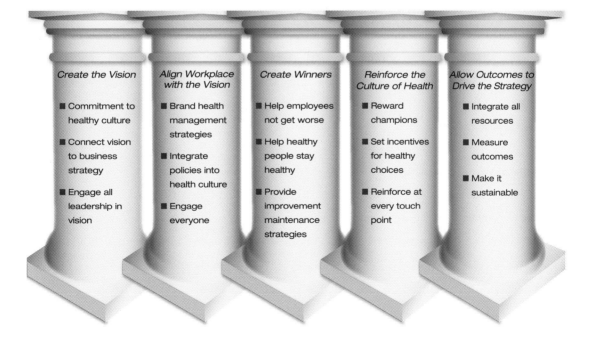

Create the Vision	Align Workplace with the Vision	Create Winners	Reinforce the Culture of Health	Allow Outcomes to Drive the Strategy
■ Commitment to healthy culture	■ Brand health management strategies	■ Help employees not get worse	■ Reward champions	■ Integrate all resources
■ Connect vision to business strategy	■ Integrate policies into health culture	■ Help healthy people stay healthy	■ Set incentives for healthy choices	■ Measure outcomes
■ Engage all leadership in vision	■ Engage everyone	■ Provide improvement maintenance strategies	■ Reinforce at every touch point	■ Make it sustainable

"Informed business leaders realize that investing in employee health results in improved productivity and long-term cost savings. The aging of the workforce, combined with a younger generation of new employees, who are less healthy than their predecessors, presents new challenges that will require thoughtful approaches to improving and maintaining employee health status. Successful approaches will be based on integrated and data-driven health and productivity programs and services."

—*Ron Finch, EdD*
Vice President
National Business Group on Health

This five pillar strategy is designed to (1) drive the vision from senior and strategic leadership level; (2) create a supportive environment via the operations leadership; (3) formulate the objectives through employee self-leadership; (4) reward and encourage positive actions that promote health management; and, (5) provide quality assurance measures for the purpose of assessing and improving the success of the effort. The strategy has the potential to engage the total population and enable companies, individuals, and families to capture the total value of health.

Four Levels of Organizational Engagement to Implement the Pillars

Not all worksites will be ready or able to implement all the concepts in this book, so we have identified four levels of commitment that reflect the engagement of company. Commitment by senior leaders and their ability to propel the process determines the appropriate engagement level for each organization. The engagement levels are do-nothing, traditional, comprehensive, and champion. Additional details about the commitment for each of the engagement levels can be found in each of the following five chapters.

Level Zero: Do Nothing

The strategy "wait for people to get sick and then try to treat them" has been in existence since companies began paying for health benefits. The strategy is driven by the medical field's obsession with reductionism, which leads research to ever-increasing, more expensive levels. The do-nothing strategy has poised us for personal and corporate bankruptcy, failure, and poor health. It cannot continue.

Table 9. Primary Features of the Do-Nothing (Wait for Sickness) Strategy

1. Benefit design focused on reducing costs
2. Prevailing philosophy is that "health is not our business"

Level One: Traditional

Currently, the majority of corporate wellness programs fall into this engagement category. They focus primarily on high-risk individuals who are sometimes defined as having a single high-risk factor. The interventions center around risk reduction and individual behavior change.

Table 10. Primary Features of Level One: Traditional Strategy

1. Benefit design focused on cost reduction
2. Traditional health promotion strategies
a. Risk reduction strategies
b. Annual HRAs
c. Onsite screening and counseling
d. Telephone coaching for high-risk individuals
e. Web-based health portal
f. Nurse advice line
g. Newsletters
h. Changes in vending machines and cafeterias
i. Wellness classes
j. Some measurement activities

Level Two: Comprehensive

A few companies recognize that the major economic gain is in helping the low-risk people stay low risk. In doing so, they increase the number of offerings including expanded coaching and measurement activities.

"A large number of employers say they have health promotion programs, but in reality, only a small minority of employers have the types of comprehensive programs and evidence-based interventions necessary to achieve a positive impact on health and dollars."

—Ron Z. Goetzel, PhD
Research Professor and Director
Institute for Health and Productivity Studies, Emory University

Table 11. Primary Features of a Comprehensive Strategy

1. Contains all of the components of the Level One programming
2. Invites employees to form a wellness committee
3. Adds some emphasis on low-risk maintenance
4. Adds coaching (either phone, Web, or e-mail) for low-risk individuals
5. Integrates resources and more intense health counseling
6. Adds more measurement activities to connect program participation to outcomes
7. Begins to engage senior management in endorsing the programs

"Too often companies look at wellness as just another benefit. We have fully integrated wellness into every aspect of our company's culture. It's a source of pride and reflects how we care for one another. As a result, wellness has become a critical element of our success."

—Steve Burd
Chairman, President, and CEO
Safeway, Inc.

Level Three: Champion Company

Level Three is the ultimate level of organizational engagement that will keep a company viable in these world-wide competitive markets. The Champion Company incorporates the five fundamental pillars to support a culture of health.

Table 12. Primary Features of Level Three: Champion Company Strategy

1. **Contains all of the components of Levels One and Two programming**

2. **Emphasizes the role of senior leadership in creating the vision**

   a. Vision connected to company strategy and people

   b. Senior leadership is visible and committed

   c. Senior leadership delegates and then transitions to cheerleaders

3. **Emphasizes the role of operations leadership in impacting the culture**

   a. Brings integrated health policies into alignment with a healthy culture

   b. Brings all policies and procedures into alignment with a healthy culture

   c. Modifies benefit design to focus on company values

   d. Integrates management of disease, crises, absence, disability and workers' compensation, and other resources

   e. Emphasizes branding of the program and direct marketing to the employee

   f. Encourages meetings with all managers and employees to manage expectations

   g. Provides incentives for all, including the low-risk individuals

4. **Emphasizes self-leadership**

   a. Provides for a health assessment system, including coaching and wellness activities for all

   b. Provides educational programs for understanding of the value of health management to the company and to the employee

   c. Offers appropriate resources to all employees, including dependents, if possible

5. **Emphasizes rewarding positive behaviors and developing the culture of health**

   a. Rewards the champions

   b. Cultivates individual respect, care, and growth

   c. Corporate culture emphasizes an abundance mentality that engages the total population

6. **Engages in quality assurance activities to get to results-driven programming**

   a. Understands the distinction between data, measurement, information, and decision support

   b. Tracks the percent of total population engaged and the percent of the total population at low risk

   c. Compares the program results with the expected natural flow of risks and costs

   d. Tracks employee and company satisfaction indicators

   e. Examines the trends of the relevant outcome measures

Assessing Organizational Engagement

The experience of our Corporate Consortium members and other companies found in the literature validates that results are related to the level of organizational engagement. Engagement at the champion level is necessary if any one company, regardless of size (small, medium or large) wants to obtain all the health and productivity benefits of a culture of health. The characteristics of each of the four levels of engagement are described above. In the subsequent chapters we provide even more detail.

In Table 13, we present a simple matrix to assess organizational engagement. The results of this assessment should help companies manage expectations related to the outcome criteria. That is, if the company engages at a traditional level, then the rewards should be expected at that same level (see Table 28 on page 165). During an early planning stage, the organizational engagement level could be selected and then the commitments required for each of the five pillars could be reviewed. It is possible that the planning team would first review the requirement within each pillar prior to selecting an engagement level for the company.

Table 13. Program Rating by Engagement Level Per Pillar

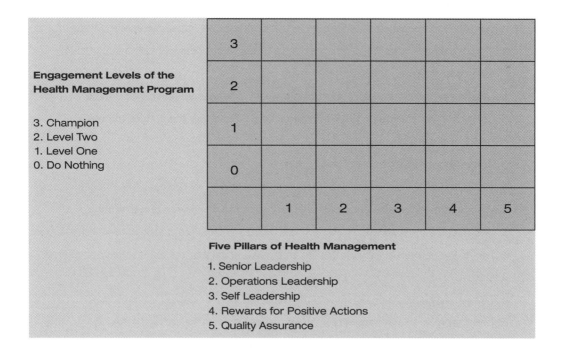

Engagement Levels of the Health Management Program

3. Champion
2. Level Two
1. Level One
0. Do Nothing

Five Pillars of Health Management

1. Senior Leadership
2. Operations Leadership
3. Self Leadership
4. Rewards for Positive Actions
5. Quality Assurance

Predicted Outcomes for the Four Levels of Organizational Engagement

In 2002, a major manufacturing company asked us to create a next generation health management program, in which they would add components progressively and advance through the four levels of commitment. We drew from the company's own six years of experience along with the best practices and outcomes from our Corporate Consortium members. We benefited from knowing the efficacy of each of these programs, plus the overall health status and economic outcomes of all of the companies where we utilized their sustainable experiences. We combined these results with our longitudinal research findings to create a modeling system that could project the expected results from the four levels of engagement: Do-Nothing, Traditional, Comprehensive, and Champion Company. Their interest, and ours, was in the health status of the total population, including the percent at low risk and the economic savings (from medical and pharmaceuticals combined) that could be achieved by helping those at low risk maintain that status.

Figure 26 shows the results of the four levels of engagement on the percent of the population at low risk over four years. The programs get progressively better as the level of engagement gets

Figure 26. Predicted Results of the Four Levels of Engagement
(Percent of Low Risk Following Each Strategy)

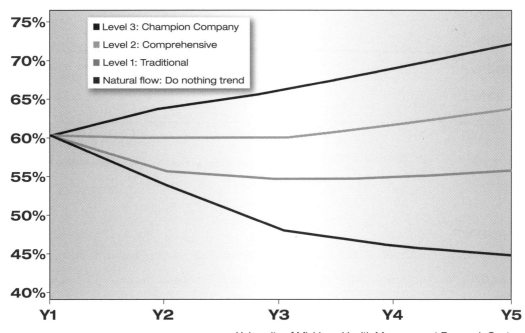

University of Michigan Health Management Research Center

higher. Level Two is typically described in the literature as a comprehensive program. Our modeling shows that it is the champion company level of engagement that moves the population to our targeted 75 percent low-risk standard. At Level Three: Champion Company, a company begins to beat the natural flow by gradually decreasing risk levels.

In addition to keeping as many employees as possible at low risk, companies are naturally interested in the economic outcomes. Figure 27 shows the savings in modeled medical and pharmaceutical expenditures over a four-year period. Each of the three intervention levels is shown to produce positive results (gross savings) but only the Champion Company achieves a zero trend outcome. The estimated cost for each program level is presented in Chapter 11.

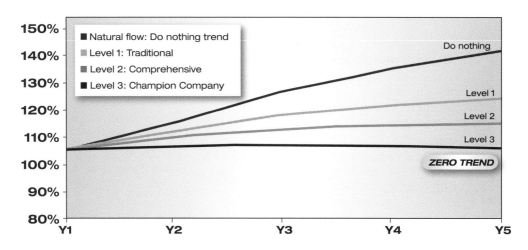

Figure 27. **Engagement Leads to Zero Trend**
(Projected Total Healthcare Costs)

University of Michigan Health Management Research Center

Viewpoint

Michael Parkinson, MD, President of the American College of Preventive Medicine, puts this in a slightly different framework that reflects the essential pillars image:

"Successful employers, those that optimize the health and productivity of their workforce (and their families), to coin a military term, deploy a 'pincer movement' strategy using highly visible 'top down' and 'bottom up' tactics.

"*Top down* includes a clear and articulate statement of where we're going and why we must change. Leaders exhibit desired personal and attitudinal behaviors which have been shown to be associated with improved health and performance—or they don't lead. Benefit programs, promotion policies, awards programs, and similar 'touch points' are aligned to reward the same behaviors. A culture is created when leaders know what is 'the expected or desired behavior' before being told.

"*Bottom up* includes empowering, truly listening to and respecting the realities of the employee and their families so that needs are met—even needs that may not be seen immediately as medical or health-related. Small successes are celebrated openly and frequently—because they are the *condicio sine qua non* of large successes."

Before initiating any of these strategies, it's important to think through the processes outlined in this chapter. Planning is a prerequisite to shaping a vision of the essential steps for success. We have observed too many false starts and sometimes failures because adequate time was not devoted to a full top-to-bottom commitment within the entire company population. The process is relatively simple:

- Decide on the basic premises on which to build the strategy and to incorporate health into the culture of the company.
- Outline the various roles and processes for each facet of the five fundamental pillars of success: senior strategic leadership, operations leadership, population self-leadership, rewards for positive behaviors, and quality assurance measures to sustain the culture of health.
- Decide at which engagement level you want to pursue your health management program.

Final Word

"When vision, strategy, tactics, metrics, and incentives are aligned transformation occurs. But it all begins person by person—'walking the talk.'"
—*Michael D. Parkinson, MD, MPH, FACPM*
President
American College of Preventive Medicine

Chapter 8: *Senior Leadership Creates the Vision*

First Fundamental Pillar to Support the Health Management Strategy

"In 2004, we launched a simple yet dynamic Dow Health Strategy that took our business case for health investment to the next level. This strategy is sharply focused on improving Dow's financial position by the promotion of better health, and features tough goals and clear metrics to ensure forward progress. Our top two priorities are prevention and quality and effectiveness of healthcare."

—Andrew N. Liveris
Chairman and CEO
The Dow Chemical Company

Vision and Engagement Starts from the Top

Any strategy to improve employee health status must have the support of senior management. In any organization (public or private, profit or nonprofit, large or small), corporate and union executives have to work together to define a clear vision of a healthy and productive workplace and workforce. Senior strategic leadership must connect the vision to the company's mission and share that vision, including the evidence that supports it, with everyone in the workforce.

"Vision without action is a daydream.
Action without vision is a nightmare."
—Japanese Proverb

In addition to integrating the vision of a healthy and productive workplace and workforce into the company culture, senior leaders must make it compatible with core business and union objectives, and share the vision with employees and their communities.

For example, suppose it has been part of the company culture to expect–even encourage–salaried employees to put in 60- or 70-hour work weeks. A manager must be empowered to buck that tradition if helping employees achieve a healthy balance between work and family responsibilities is core to the company's mission. However, for this to succeed, senior management's commitment to change has to pervade the whole organization. To be credible, a company's policies and procedures must align with the corporate mission and objectives.

"Our philosophy of employee productivity is rooted in choice and individual development. People who make better choices in their own lives will make better decisions on the job."

—*Duncan Highsmith*
Chairman
Highsmith, Inc.

Sharing the business case for a healthy and productive culture with employees is an important part of the process, and the employees need to feel that they are partners in this enterprise. The "business case" could be as simple as "it is the right thing to do" or it could utilize the evidence presented earlier to construct a full analysis of the personal benefits to individuals and the financial benefit to the company. And, companies should be transparent about the goals they set for improving the health and productivity of employees, the labor unions, and the company. Explaining that health is good for the bottom line is fine—employees want their companies to thrive. But it must be clear that the strategy is such that what's good for the business is good for employees as well. When people come to work full of energy, they are likely not only to give their best, but also draw upon that energy and motivation to carry out tasks, responsibilities, and even leisure activities in areas of their lives outside of work.

"A healthy, engaged, and productive workforce is critical to maximizing business performance and driving sustainable growth."

—*Dean Oestreich*
President
Pioneer Hi-Bred International, Inc.

In short, it seems obvious that investing time and resources for integrating health into the culture of a company is smart for any CEO. The health and productivity of the workforce is not merely an asset; it is crucial to survival. Healthcare costs are the second-biggest line item in a company's budget, after salary and wage expenses, and that doesn't even take into consideration costs associated with time away from work and time lost at work.

"Several years ago, Caterpillar recognized the impact that healthcare costs could have on our business and took action to design a long-term, sustainable healthcare plan for our employees and their families. Our new healthcare plan design encourages consumerism and the responsible use of healthcare, while putting primary focus on prevention. We will continue to take a proactive approach when it comes to employee health while still serving the needs of our business."

—Jim Owens
Chairman and CEO
Caterpillar, Inc.

However, leading the charge can be a burden for upper management. Many corporations tell Ben R. Leedle, Jr., CEO of Healthways, Inc., a health enhancement services company based in Nashville, that they don't consider it a priority to worry about the health of their employees; they want to run their businesses.

CEOs are thinking about products, profitability, shareholder value, global competition, and more. Their dance cards are full, explains Andy Webber, President of the National Business Coalition on Health, an organization that represents more than 50 healthcare business coalitions around the country. Yet he believes, "a lot of the enlightened employers are saying, 'Look, the health and productivity of my workforce is a business imperative, a competitive asset. And yes, I'm paying for healthcare, but job number 1 is to keep my workforce healthy and productive and on the job and with great vitality because that will accrue to my benefit as a business enterprise. It's a fundamental fact that I need healthy and productive workers.'"

"At Intel, prevention and wellness are a priority. Intel saves on healthcare costs, and our employees and their families get engaged in managing their health for the rest of their lives. We hear from employees every day how much they appreciate this approach. By working together, we're making a difference in both employee health and the health of Intel."

—*Paul S. Otellini*
President and CEO
Intel Corporation

Many corporate leaders grasp the business case for investing in the health and well-being of their employees, but they don't necessarily take a personal interest in seeing the changes through. What has to happen, Ben Leedle insists, is for CEOs to wake up each morning asking themselves, "What can I do today to create an environment that leads to the healthiest and most productive workforce possible?"

We're committed to engaging our Associates in making healthy choices for themselves and their families, with the goal of maintaining their health and well-being. Ultimately, a healthy workforce is good for our Associates, communities, customers, and business."

—*H. Lee Scott, Jr.*
President and CEO
Wal-Mart Stores, Inc.

At Healthways, making sure that their 4,000+ employees and their families meet their individual health goals is especially important. Healthways employees apply what they learn about achieving optimum health status to helping other businesses do the same for their employees. Leedle believes that each individual should have three supportive environments–a medical home, a personal home, and a work home that all promote good health. Healthways is defining what the environment of that healthy work home can look like. Ben Leedle is right in the thick of that environment, exercising and striving to lose weight right alongside his fellow employees.

"The people who can do the most to fix America's healthcare crisis in the next three to five years are business leaders."

—Ben R. Leedle, Jr.
President and CEO
Healthways, Inc.

It is not enough for top executives simply to approve the idea of a health management program and then step back and expect others to implement it. Support for the health and well-being of employees has to be incorporated into the values of the organization, and that can only come from the top. Without a comprehensive, clear, shared vision, even the most viable program is susceptible to losing momentum and eventually disintegrating.

Crown Equipment in New Bremen, Ohio is a good example, "We started HealthWise, a health and productivity management program, in 2004 with a HealthWise manager, a HealthWise committee, and support from our medical director. We also worked closely with health partners outside of our company," says President Jim Dicke III. "To track the progress of our program, we developed key measurements. The good news is that more than 90 percent of Crown employees and eligible spouses in the United States participate in the program each year. In addition, the percentage of our employees in the low risk category has significantly increased and we have already seen improvement in our medical costs per employee."

Dicke also notes key elements that have contributed to the success of the HealthWise Program including a health benefit credit for participation, health advisers for all employees and spouses, ongoing support from the University of Michigan Health Management Research Center, and the commitment of senior management to good health. Dicke considers the HealthWise Program a win-win situation and an integral part of Crown's success.

The challenge to senior leadership, then, is to put the systems for a healthy culture in place. What does a healthy and productive organization look like? Creating the vision is not necessarily an easy task, and every senior manager has to be part of the process.

"The spirit of the organization is created from the top."

—Peter Drucker
1909–2005

Moving from a Vision to Change Action

The degree of commitment at the highest level is the first step that transforms strategy into reality. This first step is often missing. Unless this support is highly visible and becomes part of the mainstream of decision making, some programs never achieve sustainability. Successful programs confirm that a well-defined vision is the first step in transitioning worksite health promotion from an idealistic vision to a serious business strategy.

King County (which includes Seattle) in the State of Washington, has been successful in holding increases in healthcare costs to among the lowest in public sector organizations across the country. At the same time they have resisted cost shifting to employees, despite a great pressure to do so. Ron Sims, King County Executive explains their philosophy and strategy as, "Sustained improvement for the long haul requires change on both the supply and demand sides of the healthcare equation. On the demand side, employees must feel that they have a larger role to play in their own health outcomes. That means giving them the tools for engagement and a very supportive environment at work. On the supply side we have to shine a light on the practices and performance of our healthcare delivery system, in order to measure and reward for quality outcomes.

"I refuse to accept the conventional 'first options' of cutting benefits and shifting costs. These strategies may buy you a year or two, but they just put off a terrible day of financial reckoning.

"With over 90 percent participation, Healthy Incentives^{SM} is the fulcrum for building our culture of wellness at King County. Once our plan members know where they stand health wise, they're far more ready to engage in their own well-being, both at home and at work.

"The first move is always the hardest. The programs and policies at King County's Health Reform Initiative are designed to build a culture of wellness in the workplace, to break down the patterns of isolation that keep people from making that critical decision—to act.

"All the vision in the world won't get you to the promised land of sustained reform. It takes leadership by example, if you expect your employees to embrace change."

Another example of the senior executive leading change is in Jackson, Michigan, where Georgia Fojtasek, CEO and President of Allegiance Health System, realized that increases in healthcare dollars were going to stretch local business too far for them to survive. Although she realized that health systems can make a lot of money solely treating the sick, she also realized a community obligation. "Our top leadership had to believe in this effort in order for us to budget for it and fund it. We started with our own employees and six volunteer companies in the community and now we have expanded into a true community effort. We have spent on average probably $3 million per year out of the system's reserves since 2000. So we had to look at it as a long-term business investment and

I think that if you don't have top leadership who believe, then the programs are going to be subject to discontinuation when the financial challenges start, which they will."

No subsequent step can override the lack of a serious commitment from senior leadership. To achieve success, the vision has to be clear, connected to company strategy, shared with employees, supported by other upper management, and union leaders, and turned over to operations for implementation. (See Table 14) Only then can senior leadership take on the cheerleader role.

"When a company's leaders make it a priority to address the underlying causes of poor health and high healthcare costs, they reap the rewards. They see an increase in productivity, output, retention and creative energy. At the same time, they achieve lower healthcare costs than their peer companies. An executive may not view this as healthcare reform, but it is."

—John Clymer
Former President
Partnership for Prevention

Table 14. **Vision from the Senior Leadership**

- Clear vision within leadership

- Vision connected to company strategy

- Vision shared with employees

- Accountability and responsibility assigned to operations leadership

- Leadership of the company and unions transition to become the cheerleaders

Delegating for Implementation

Next, senior leadership has to delegate responsibility to operations leadership to oversee the program's implementation. This process, which includes delegating appropriate responsibility and accountability, is key to ensuring that the work environment, including all benefit designs and all policies and procedures, are aligned with the vision. This step ensures that the vision is implemented at every level within the organization and that every employee has an opportunity to engage. Management will have to decide on the use of incentives to involve all employees and, if possible, their family members, and to keep them engaged throughout the year. Finally, senior leaders will have to become cheerleaders of the new strategy; cheerleaders within the company and cheerleaders of the company's strategy to reach outside the community.

Managers entrusted with engaging the employee population in the health management program know too well the importance of support from senior leadership. Paula Sauer, Manager of the program for Medical Mutual of Ohio, knows that the late Kent Clapp, CEO and Chairman, was a major supporter and often was seen in the cafeteria or screening sessions talking with employees about the program (Note: unfortunately Kent died in a plane crash in the fall of 2008). "You've got to have executive support. You've got to have dedicated human resources that work on wellness, and you've got to have financial resources. And that's where I see the biggest holes in the market. If the chairman doesn't support it, you are not going to be successful. If the CFO doesn't support it financially, you are not going to be successful. And if this is one little piece of the HR person's job, you are not going to be successful. It is a total team effort with strong commitments."

"Many CEOs and CFOs are realizing the benefits of investing in their human capital. The key to implementation success is getting the CEO to set health enhancement as a vision and clearly educate middle management that this is a major corporate initiative. One of the best ways to achieve this is to give middle management and the HR department annual merit and salary increases based partly on the achievement of corporate wellness goals and objectives."

—David Rearick, DO, MBA
Vice President of Medical Management
Strategic Benefit Solutions

Summary and Ranking to Reach Champion Company Level

As evidenced by the ranking categories in Table 15, we think the only way to get to Champion Level in the leadership and vision category is to have a clear vision connected to the business strategy, shared with all employees, and have senior management (company and union) clearly visible in the implementation of the vision.

Table 15. Engagement Levels for Senior Leadership

Leadership Commitment and Vision	Do Nothing	Level One	Level Two	Champion Company
1. Adequate funding for engagement level	X	X	X	X
2. Assign responsibility for implementation		X	X	X
3. Vision of a healthy and productive company			X	X
a. Consistent with business strategy				X
b. Decisions based on gap analyses				X
c. Agreed upon by leadership				X
d. Shared with employees				X
e. Remains highly visible				X
f. Active as a participant and as a cheerleader				X
4. Engagement by managers and leaders at all levels				X
5. Transition to cheerleaders				X

Final Word

"People look to the top to see what's important. When leaders include health and well-being as a major strategic initiative and are serious about it, good things happen."

—Margie Blanchard, PhD
Co-Founder, Former President and CEO
The Ken Blanchard Companies

Chapter 9: *Operations Leadership Implements the Vision*

Second Fundamental Pillar to Support the Health Management Strategy

*"Our goal is to help employees perform at the top of their game at work,
at home and into retirement."*

—Dan Ustain
Chairman, President, and CEO
Navistar International Corporation

Fixing the Missed Opportunity

When we first began work in this field, we assumed our focus was going to be the health of the workforce. We believed that the sequence would look like this: health management programs would influence healthier lifestyles, which would lead to healthy people who would then become better employees, which would bring about gains for the organization. We then went about our research work in a systematic way to produce the best possible business case.

Health Promotion Intervention—Healthy People—Better Employees— Gains for the Organization

In the purpose and design of our studies, we constructed a business case that meets the demands of the corporate world. The business case is built upon the organization's ability to retain and move others to low-risk behaviors. When companies asked how to do this, we pointed them in the direction of risk reduction interventions. Subsequently, we learned that individual risk reduction intervention strategies alone are basically ineffective. Upon examination, we found that participation levels were extremely low, and that significant change in the organization was not possible. In addition, we looked at the recidivism data and learned that even if a risk reduction program were successful in persuading individuals to change, they relapsed after returning to the same work environment.

We could have predicted those results. The basic flaw in the risk reduction strategy is that the health promotion professionals failed to factor in how the high-risk people became high risk in the first place. And, they did not consider how to keep those individuals low risk even if they did achieve behavior change.

The second basic flaw was the absence of an intervention that would keep low- risk people at low risk. Finally, we realized that the key to success was to modify the workplace culture to support a healthy and productive population. As one of the training directors at General Electric's Leadership Development Center at Crotonville in New York State noted,

"You never send a changed person back to an unchanged environment."

Operations Leadership—Align the Workplace with the Vision

The challenge to the operations leadership is to create an environment within the company that convinces low-risk individuals to remain low risk, as well as supporting the high-risk individuals in making sustainable behavior changes. Operations managers have the external and internal resources to integrate health successfully into their company culture. Consistent with the way we have seen many organizations begin to think about possibilities and options, we have organized this chapter into three parts.

"Goals get people going. Values sustain the efforts."
—Ken Blanchard
Co-Founder and Chief Spiritual Officer
The Ken Blanchard Companies

Part 1 is a review of the important roles, contributions, and best advice and products of the external partners, which include health plans, primary care physicians, pharmaceutical companies—seven categories in all, which are detailed in the section that follows. Obviously, the health and productivity of the workplace and the workforce is too important to be left solely to the external partners or even to the selected healthcare benefit plan. Part 2 is a discussion of how internal management can make health an integral part of the organization's core culture, and in Part 3, we discuss the role of operations leadership in making this happen.

"When we study best practices, what emerges as a key success factor is active senior leadership commitment and engagement. Health promotion programs can't be seen as being under the radar screen. They have to become part and parcel of the organization's fabric and culture."

—Ron Z. Goetzel, PhD
Research Professor and Director
Institute for Health and Productivity Studies, Emory University

Part 1: Transformation of the External Partners

When the CEO and other senior leaders provide a vision for a healthy and productive company, with every decision taking the well-being of employees into account, integrative health strategies become an important part of the company culture. To help that evolution take place, CEOs, their senior leaders, and the operations leadership are turning to an increasing number of partners for help. Creating a culture that facilitates health and productivity is of such great importance that nearly all companies need to seek expert guidance and support.

Companies work with at least seven major categories of partners:

1. **Health plans**
2. **Benefit consultants**
3. **Primary care physicians**
4. **Pharmaceutical companies**
5. **Health enhancement companies**
6. **Health systems**
7. **Community and state governments**

What's most important is that businesses work with these experts as partners, rather than vendors. Vendors don't share an organization's economic or business goals, and companies can't afford to have noncommittal relationships when so much is at stake. Partners, on the other hand, do share a commitment and common goals. When one succeeds, the other succeeds and when one makes a profit, the other makes a profit.

For too long companies had resigned themselves to paying for just healthcare without asking for any improvement in quality or a cooperative working environment. When Steelcase was adding an enhancement to its existing and successful wellness program, Director of Benefits Marshall Beard called a meeting of all of the healthcare providers (stakeholders) that served Steelcase's employees and their families. One of his introductory comments was, "…we enjoy working with each of you as we have in the past and to maintain that partnership, here is what we want you to do…" He set the tone for a climate of cooperation with Steelcase and with each other. Steelcase was an early example of a company sharing its vision with its vendors and turning them into partners.

Health plans

American companies are tired of paying for healthcare that covers only sick care. Look at what decades of paying has achieved: spiraling costs and increasing rates of poor health and chronic illnesses. No other supplier, vendor, or partner would have survived even six months with that record. Companies are now asking insurance companies to add wellness care to their product lines, or better yet, roll a wellness component into their current plans with no increase in cost. Responsive insurance companies are doing that, now, and in the process are transitioning into comprehensive "health services plans" rather than traditional "insurance companies." The insurance companies that continue to only pay only for sickness care may be destined to go out of business.

"Improve health. It's our single focus. It means we stand for care that's effective and personal choices that matter. It means we connect the health of your employees to the health of your business."

—*David Cordani*
President and COO
CIGNA Corporation

Health plans are in a unique position to help companies actively promote health to an overall employee population as well as spouses and dependents. Stand-alone or disease-specific programs often influence individuals with specific health concerns, but champion company level health plans are positioned to reach the total population. They have the capacity to provide a continuum of care, from wellness services to care management to disease management, and they can aid in the return-to-work process. Further, health plans have access to data that identifies the best physicians and health systems based on cost and quality.

"Encouraging a healthy lifestyle makes sense for everyone. At Aetna, it's our business to invest in programs to help employees stay healthy and be their best, at work and at home. It's clear that encouraging a healthy lifestyle makes good business sense."

—*John W. Rowe, MD*
Chairman and CEO
Aetna, Inc.

Health plans are increasingly working with employers to achieve champion company level health management goals—some are even guaranteeing results. A number of health plans are reshaping their own business plans to include a focus on keeping healthy people healthy. These plans aren't shirking the financial tasks of paying for physician and hospital services, but are expanding their mission to help people achieve and maintain their optimum level of health.

"Healthcare purchasers of all sizes are recognizing the very real and measurable business value of investing in a culture of health," says Peter Roberts, President of Wellmark Blue Cross and Blue Shield. "What started as a narrow focus on wellness has now evolved to include employee policies and procedures, environmental factors, work-life balance, stress management, and a host of other factors influencing employees and their families each and every day."

"To successfully help healthcare purchasers build a culture of health over time, insurance carriers need to expand their role beyond rating and paying acute care medical claims to becoming a true health plan and they need to redirect resources across the full spectrum of employee health."

—*Peter Roberts*
President
Wellmark Blue Cross and Blue Shield

Forward-thinking health plans bring a wide range of experience, knowledge, and tools to their partnerships with companies. At CIGNA HealthCare, researchers are working to understand the data it collects on individuals and employee populations and integrate it into the services it offers companies. Consumers polled by CIGNA say that they value their health above almost everything else. People feel lucky to be well, to not be in the hospital, and not to be facing a major disease.

But being healthy isn't luck, it's a choice. And being healthy is much more than not being sick. It is having energy, vitality, and feeling at the top of your game. "When we conduct focus groups, people say they view their health as their most important asset. But it's an asset that they take for granted until they don't have it. There's a great opportunity to help people understand their role in staying well," says H. Edward Hanway, Chairman and CEO at CIGNA.

"Our energy had traditionally been focused on the 20 percent of members who had acute or chronic health conditions. Now we are spending a significant amount of time identifying people who are healthy but at risk. If we can get them to recognize that they are at risk, and then provide services that enable them to take control of that situation, we can prevent acute and chronic conditions from developing."

—H. Edward Hanway
Chairman and CEO
CIGNA Corporation

CIGNA studies its data—everything from HRA (health risk appraisal) results to pharmacy, medical, disability, and behavioral claims—and then develops company-specific programs based on that information. Many health plans also draw on the data and services of their subsidiaries to offer more comprehensive wellness programs. When CIGNA puts together programs, it takes information from its expanded Health Solutions unit (formerly behavioral health) into account. It also relies on services supported by that area to bolster its overall health management initiatives. Keeping a member well after a heart attack, for example, includes screening for depression. It is known now that if depression goes undiagnosed and untreated, people face a much higher probability of a second heart attack.

Health plans are striving to add health management services to their traditional disease care focus. Optum Health, a subsidiary of United Healthcare provides a comprehensive population based program to its clients by combining wellness and mental health services to form a continuum of care. Approaches to health management programming are becoming more sophisticated, and they cover a spectrum of care, according to Camille Haltom, National Vice President for Consultant Relations for Optum Health and United Health Group. They have programs for all employees and their family members, whether they are healthy, living with illness, or facing a need for intensive care.

"In the '80s, employers who had wellness programs focused mostly on fitness. What has evolved is a focus on helping people to optimize their health and well-being. It's a much broader stroke and it appeals to individuals regardless of where they sit on the healthcare continuum. There is something for every part of the population."

—Camille Haltom
National Vice President for Consultant Relations
Optum Health and United Health Group

Health plans are also natural partners in the goal of creating a healthy community. Medical Mutual of Ohio launched a three-year effort to support the health of residents in the Cleveland suburb of Solon, where the city government, the school system, and several businesses are clients. The community has generated a high level of excitement by promoting wellness through health fairs, marketing efforts and local restaurant participation. Area companies are direct beneficiaries of this initiative since this is where their workforce lives. The community may turn out to be just as important as the company in encouraging a healthy and productive quality of life.

"Insurance companies are encouraging employers to offer more aggressive wellness programs to their employees. Health plans are even guaranteeing results, putting their fees at risk if a population doesn't meet clinical outcomes," says Jack Bastable, National Practice Leader for Health and Productivity Management at CBIZ Benefits & Insurance Services. "That's huge for insurers. Recently, I was in a room with an actuary who told my clients that the single most important thing their companies could do to impact their claims, their utilization, and their cost increases was to help their employees stay healthy. That wasn't a marketing person, a salesperson, or a physician. It was an actuary."

History will show that the evolution from insurance companies to health plans is one of the most transformational movements of our times.

Health Enhancement Companies

A whole new industry has grown up around health management. Health enhancement organizations, which provide services directly to employers or as part of a health plan's offerings, have the expertise to help individuals move toward a higher health status via risk reduction. Many of these companies have had years of experience; they've learned what works and what doesn't. They are able to tailor programs to meet an employer's specific goals. "The number of health promotion companies has grown fairly large," says Michael O'Donnell, PhD, MBA, MPH, Editor-in-Chief, and President of the *American Journal of Health Promotion.* "The primary cause of the growth is uncontrollable healthcare costs that are consuming more than 16 percent of our GDP and are expected to grow to 20 percent in a decade. Fortunately, we have a growing body of evidence that shows health promotion programs can reduce medical costs and improve people's health. The field is already taking off, but my prediction is that it's going to grow at least tenfold."

"Enlightened, sophisticated employers see health management not as an operating cost but an investment in workforce health and productivity."

—*Andy Webber*
President
National Business Coalition on Health

Experience is helping the Nashville-based firm Healthways to assist clients—and their employees—to broaden the way they think about health management, both in the programs they offer and the benefits they realize. "We've learned that if we can get people interested in health in one aspect of their life, it's easier to get them thinking about other healthy behaviors," explains Healthways' Vice President and Chief Medical Officer Dexter Shurney. "So helping someone quit smoking can lead to discussions about healthy eating and reducing stress. In the same way, each healthy behavior has many useful connections. Most employers understand that exercise reduces an individual's cardiovascular risk. But they may not realize that it also increases metabolism, decreases a person's risk for stress and depression, and helps a person sleep better."

Shurney envisions a time when a company's focus on health is so ingrained in its culture that no one would dream of bringing donuts to an early-morning meeting. He explains: "An organization in the future might share the healthcare cost savings it achieves with its employees. That might make it very taboo for employees to live unhealthy lifestyles. They would be accountable to their colleagues."

"It doesn't need to be punitive," he adds. "An employee might ask an office mate to join him on a walk over lunchtime. It becomes part of the culture, and the culture would not support unhealthy choices. So in the new culture everyone is going to say, 'When we have a business meeting, don't bring donuts for breakfast. We know better than this. That's not helping us or the organization.'"

"New tools, models, and theories arise every few years. Yet the fundamentals of health management remain the same: Providing a healthy work environment, along with resources for individuals to take responsibility for their health, results in sustainable population health management and a competitive advantage. Our goal as a partner with organizations is to develop the best resources for helping individuals and organizations improve health."

—*Dean Witherspoon*
President
Health Enhancement Systems

Whatever approaches an employer and a health enhancement company designs will be based on the mutual need to succeed, Shurney believes. The heightened interest in wellness is creating an opportunity for these companies. "But we have to get it right," Shurney says. "If we get it wrong, it could set us back several years." That's the motivation of a partner.

Health coaching is an example where managing expectations is crucial to the success of the coaching experience. Operations leadership or an outside health enhancement company must set the stage for the coaching program, as a part of the health risk appraisal system. Janet Walker, through her experience with the Achieva Lifetime Health (acquired by CIGNA Health Services), says that, "Onsite presentations, ideally given by health coaches, can help prepare participants for the initial contact and therefore make the sessions that much more meaningful. Employers can facilitate the onsite presentations by health coaches, which can help prepare participants for what to expect from the process."

At WellSteps, Vice President Troy Adams says, "We have learned that there are two factors critical to the success of health and productivity management initiatives: culture change and behavior change. It is easier for employees to adopt and maintain healthy behaviors in a supportive culture, therefore, things like healthy food options, opportunities to be physically active, and smoking policy really matter! We have also learned that communicating personal risk status and providing consumer health education are simply not enough to prompt behavior change. Employees are more likely to attempt a behavior change when they are invited, guided, and given a compelling reason to try."

Companies like Summit Health, Medifit, and Health Solutions add considerable value to more comprehensive health companies through their excellence in providing health risk appraisals and biometric screenings. These companies are especially valuable for clients with multi-site locations, sometimes spread throughout the country. The can get the same material and testing quality to each employee and family member regardless of location.

Another health enhancement company, StayWell Health Management, has been in business serving the employer market continuously since 1978. David Anderson, Senior Vice President and Chief Health Officer, believes they have been providing services longer than any other commercial vendor and feels they have come a tremendous distance in the past 30 years. The pace of change is accelerating. "We've established that well-designed, well implemented health management strategies are effective in improving health in a cost-effective manner, and we have a reasonable case for a positive return on investment.

"While wellness programs are the norm for employers, less than five percent incorporate the range of best practices we know are critical for optimal results. These programs report positive impacts on health and on healthcare and productivity-related costs, and these solid results are being realized despite the fact that many 'best-practice' programs are still less than optimal. In a recent study, StayWell found that only 50 percent the best-practice companies we examined had strong management support for their wellness program. And nothing so profoundly affects the potential for creating a culture of wellness at the worksite as senior leadership that embraces health as a core business value. Well-managed human capital yields competitive advantage, and few things affect the performance of employees as profoundly as their health. Embracing health as a core business value opens all doors for the wellness program."

"I have been in this business for years, and I've never seen this level of interest—ever. Things have changed. People understand that the lifestyle we are living as a society is really driving health risks and that there is a definite impact. People see the connection."

—Dexter Shurney, MD
Medical Director
Healthways

Benefit Consultants

Most companies use benefit consulting organizations to help them with sorting through all the intricacies of providing for the health and safety of their employees. However if the benefit consultants only provide advice around co-pays, deductibles and sickness-care coverage they are behaving more like vendors than true partners. That is, they are selling the products they have but not always the products their clients need. However, in the best case they can help companies and individuals learn about and select benefit plans that meet health management goals and bring total value to the organization.

Thomas P. McGraw, President of McGraw-Wentworth Benefit Consulting Company, working with small to mid-size companies observes, "Like other employers, small and mid-sized firms face the challenge of escalating healthcare costs. Tried and true strategies for reducing costs, such as deductible and co-pay increases, payroll contribution increases, eligibility restrictions and the like have been pursued regularly over the last several years. Employers and their employees are tired of constant plan changes.

"Recently employers have been focusing on wellness programs as a way to reduce healthcare costs. Their thinking is sound: To the degree they can improve the health status of their covered population, they can lower the need for healthcare services and, therefore, healthcare costs. Wellness programs have become more prevalent over the last five years.

"In embarking on a wellness program, employers are targeting reductions in healthcare spending first and foremost. At the same time, they understand that a wellness program may be effective at boosting productivity, improving employee loyalty and demonstrating corporate responsibility. In combination, all of these factors make wellness programs attractive."

"People really only have to answer two questions related to their healthcare: When I must access care, how do I do it efficiently, cost effectively and with the best possible outcome? And, how do I keep from needing to access care in the first place?"

—Mike Campbell
President
CLS Benefits and the Wellness Council of Indiana

Companies are actively seeking information about how to help employees stay well, and that's exciting to Barry Hall, a principal at Buck Consultants—an ACS company. Hall has believed in the potential of health management strategies for years, and he's able to share success stories from clients that have created healthier environments.

One of the reasons Hall enjoys working in this area is that it can have gains for both a company and individual employees. The key, he says, is clear communication from management to employees: "These are our health costs, they are rising, and we have to do something about it. We don't want to keep asking you to pay more, but we can't pay any more or we're going to go out of business, so here's what we need to do together."

"This is not easy, and it takes a real commitment from an employer. But when a company does make a commitment to creating a culture of health, employees respond, and it becomes all the things that we hope for: a better place to work with happier, healthier and more productive workers. The challenges are real, but so are the benefits."

—Barry Hall
Principal
Buck Consultants, an ACS company

"It's up to the company to give its employees the tools they need and an environment that keeps them well, but employees bear the responsibility to manage their health status." Hall says, "Once employees understand this and begin to participate, they feel a part of the effort to manage healthcare costs. In addition to feeling healthier, they understand that they are helping their company thrive."

For small to mid-size companies, however, Thomas McGraw says, "A crucial issue remains. How does the mid-sized firm go about measuring whether their wellness program is successful? How do they measure whether the health status of the covered population has been improved? To put it more precisely, how does the human resource director convince the CFO or CEO that the resources spent on wellness initiatives are worth the result? More work needs to be done in this area with respect to wellness programs if a compelling business case is to be presented. Regrettably, we see little analysis on the part of wellness consultants serving the mid-sized market when it comes to addressing this issue. The wellness consultant who can provide both a) best-in-class health risk assessment, biometric screening and coaching programs and, b) incisive and insightful analysis on health status improvement and, therefore, expected claim cost reduction, will have an enormous competitive advantage in the marketplace."

Primary Care Physicians

Primary care physicians are the first line of defense against sickness. People tend to trust their doctors, and health promoting cultures need to engage them, not as gatekeepers, but as an accessible resource for wellness services as well as for disease care. Primary care physicians can be a major ally in disease prevention and early detection, producing significant cost savings compared to late detection or chronic disease.

For example, one primary care physician, Gregg Stefanek, DO, has taken the initiative to partner with community organizations and businesses in Alma, Michigan. He has conducted free health screenings and free health risk assessments at several businesses, ranging from a seven-employee hardware store to Alma College, which now gives its employees an extra 15 minutes at lunch to exercise. The city-wide effort is supported by a local physician foundation, but Stefanek, who talks about wellness with every one of his own patients, believes physicians can do more.

"Primary care physicians have a responsibility to speak on wellness to large groups, to make themselves available to school boards and community healthcare task forces, and to be a resource in general to local governments and businesses that are striving to encourage and support healthy behaviors," he says.

"One area that we don't do enough of is working young people. Where is our future workforce? In high schools! High schools are seeing epidemics of obesity and poor health. So we need to focus some of our efforts on the younger generation."

—Gregg Stefanek, DO
Primary Care Physician
Alma, Michigan

Another approach that is proving effective is the "medical home," in which the company, in keeping with its benefit design and health plan, arranges for all of its employees to be under the care of one of several convenient physician or medical groups. The physician coordinates the care of the employee and family members and maintains records of tests and treatment history which are accessible by the member and specialty groups.

The idea of a medical home seems like a great innovation but there are certain issues that need to be addressed. Tehseen Salimi, MD, MHA, Senior Medical Director at sanofi-aventis, observes that most chronically ill patients in the United States do not receive care in an integrated delivery system but through a network for private practitioners operating independently in the community. "Traditionally, care coordination has been the responsibility of primary care physicians, who have the training and, generally, the motivation to do so. The requirements for coordinating care of complex patients (especially those with chronic conditions), however, are overwhelming the capacity of many primary care practices. To the frustration of primary care physicians, and their patients, it is difficult to marshal resources, direct services and intelligently share essential information in a coordinated manner to support the fulfillment of prescribed care plans. Moreover, the capital investment and practice transformation required to become eHealth capable are considerable and beyond the reach of many small practices.

"Patients today have unprecedented access to healthcare information, enabling them to more fully participate in, and assume responsibility for their care. Changes in health insurance benefit design are encouraging patients to become more engaged as informed consumers. Ancillary health-support services such as case management and disease management also are increasingly available."

IBM realized that the workplace is an essential piece of any program that encourages people to value their health. "The long-term, sustainable outcomes are driven by experiences in the healthcare system," explains Martin Sepulveda, Vice President of Global Well-Being Services and Health Benefits. Accordingly, IBM has encouraged the use of the Medical Home strategy to connect the employee with the primary care physicians and the local healthcare community. On a global scale, IBM sponsors local initiatives in many countries, including safe transportation, local medical and health services, subsidized housing, as well as many other solutions that impact the well-being for its employees.

"People's behaviors are most influenced by their care providers, and primary care physicians are one of the critical points for transformation within in the health environment."

—*Martin Sepulveda, MD*
Vice President of Global Well-Being Services and Health Benefits
IBM

Pharmaceutical Companies

Pharmaceutical companies, which originally developed drugs to treat diseases, now manufacture a growing number of medications that people need to control chronic conditions and reduce risk factors such as high blood pressure and high cholesterol. These lifestyle drugs will be in increasing demand as people change their definition of health from the absence of disease to the presence of vitality and well-being. Pharmaceutical companies have built strong health maintenance models into their products, making them natural partners in any company's effort to make health a key component of its culture.

Drug companies are also very effective at creating awareness through brand recognition and driving consumer demand through advertising, an area of expertise that can also be applied to "selling" the concept of wellness. Our challenge is to expand the pharmaceuticals' economic interests from a model based on marketing single products to one that rewards promoting a more effective health management system. Imagine a marketing campaign for overall wellness that is as powerful as advertising that creates demand for a certain medication. Condition management will be a key component to a healthcare system that emphasizes wellness care as much as sickness care, and the pharmaceutical industry plays a huge role in that area. It is becoming a part of our cultural change.

Companies are looking for ways to better communicate directly with employers, according to one executive at a pharmaceutical company. Companies are discovering that employers do not respond well to the sales pitches that appeal to physicians, nor to the mathematical models that are used with managed care companies. So to build stronger partnerships, these companies have developed tools and messages that make more sense for employers. For example, the drug firm can show healthcare cost comparisons for someone who has achieved optimal health status with someone of medium or high risk, enabling executives to build a business case for helping individuals get and stay healthy.

Companies are also partnering with businesses to educate employees. Drug firms compile reams of information about the diseases for which they are developing drugs. This research, combined with that of other pharmaceutical companies is used to create state-of-the-art teaching tools to help employees take better care of themselves.

Health Systems

Realistically, health systems which are focused on providing sickness care have few economic incentives to partner with organizations and communities in creating a culture of health. Until hospitals develop new economic models, their core need will be to maintain a high occupancy of hospital and operating room beds rather than promoting high health status for the populations they serve.

And, people will always need sickness care. Nonetheless, hospitals may, in time, also play a key role in the transformation to a culture of health.

In some communities, this is already beginning to happen. For example, in Alma, Michigan, a hospital donated laboratory resources for checking cholesterol and sugar levels when local businesses offered health screenings to their employees.

Allegiance Health, a health system in Jackson, Michigan, is at the center of a communitywide effort to help residents live healthier lives and avoid preventable illnesses. In October 2008, writer Milt Freudenheim of the New York Times highlighted the community project as well as the hospital's history of striving to provide affordable healthcare services. When the health system purchased an HMO in the late '90s and then had to raise premiums 40 percent in a single year, it began looking at data to determine what was costing so much. "We realized that it had much less to do with our provider rates than it did with per unit use," says Georgia Fojtasek, President and CEO of Allegiance Health. "We then began the journey of looking at the opportunity for impacting the actual demand of healthcare based on health status."

"People are increasingly aware of the high rates of health problems in our country, and they look to health systems to define how to make a difference. They put it under the rubric of healthcare, even though we know it's not about healthcare—it's about health."

—Georgia Fojtasek
President and CEO
Allegiance Health

Fojtasek and her management team devised a plan in which Allegiance's insurance subsidiary would partner with employers as a health improvement organization rather than a health maintenance organization. Working with six employers, Allegiance launched a program called "It's Your Life," which offers health coaching to employees. The model has been successful in reducing risks in employee populations. Allegiance also reaches out to the community in a variety of ways, and it sees value in a reputation linked to wellness. In a client survey, it seeks to answer the question: "Are we engaged in helping the community reduce healthcare costs and improve health?"

Health providers have a financial incentive to treat sick people, but Fojtasek believes that will change over time. "For now we are just going to have to figure out how to make these investments, understanding that in the early stages, reimbursement isn't likely to be there."

Communities

In addition to the above partners, there has to be help from within the broader community. As Gary Earl, Senior Vice President at CIGNA, explains, "For nearly an entire century, the focus, energies and resources of the vast collection of professionals, leaders and experts, as related to the term health have been aimed primarily at the treatment, prevention and or avoidance of illness and disease. However, despite both the individual and collective intentions and efforts to make treatments more effective and costs more manageable, by many if not most measurements, we collectively have fallen short of the mark.

"Having dedicated nearly 30 years to the world of health, health improvement, wellness, human capital and population health management, on both a personal and professional level, I am convinced by the evidence that has been uncovered and verified, that the highest hope for a sustainable, meaningful and measurable solution, or path into the challenge, as well as renewal of system we have invested in will come through a change in perspective. I believe it will come through the broadening of our combined and collective view, understanding, and appreciation for the individual's condition and behavior as connected to their social, cultural and environmental surroundings. Our greatest opportunity for success will occur by seeing the root level determinants of health as connected, related to one's opportunity to make change and thus taking action from this total view."

Community organizations such as Chambers of Commerce, fraternal groups, economic clubs, schools, faith groups, civic organizations, and others all could contribute to a healthy and productive environment. Community involvement is an important aspect of creating a culture of health. How can a healthy family or a healthy company function in an unhealthy setting? At some point, neighborhoods, cities, and states are going to have to realize and act upon the fact that a healthy and productive culture is vital to the economic future of the companies doing business within their boundaries.

Some communities are in the early stages of implementing programs aimed at helping citizens maintain and improve their health status. The Center for Health Transformation, a collaboration of private organizations and public entities founded by former House Speaker Newt Gingrich, develops and supports innovative ideas for transforming our healthcare system, and is working with several cities and states to institute programs aimed at keeping people well. In Georgia, 27 employers and all of the major insurers are working together and with the Center to systematize care for people with diabetes. Columbus, Georgia has become a model city for the "21st century healthy community." Physician leaders, employers, the Chamber of Commerce, and local health systems are all involved, according to Nancy Desmond, CEO of the Center for Health Transformation and the Gingrich Group.

"People need to understand that real change requires real change. Trying to make minor adjustments to the existing healthcare system is not going to work. We need to look at the bigger picture of where we as Americans can go. American has a great history of being innovative and moving forward."

—Nancy Desmond

CEO

Center for Health Transformation and the Gingrich Group

Another community project to follow is Building a Healthier Chicago. According to the Web site (www.healthierchicago.org) their goal is, "...to improve the health of Chicago's residents and employees through the integration of existing and new public health, medicine and community health promotion activities." The model is to build a coalition of local entities to create a system of interventions that complement and reinforce each other to maximize reach and effectiveness. The over 50 entities include health care organizations, worksites, schools, faith-based organizations, homes, and neighborhoods of Chicago.

"The foundation of success for our nation's healthcare is based on the development of a broad social movement in wellness. The new age of wellness must be grounded in the bedrock of community, in all its forms."

—James M. Galloway, MD, FACP, FAHA

Assistant U.S. Surgeon General, Acting HHS Regional Director

Region V

Summary and Engagement Scoring for External Partners

Nearly all companies have relied on these external partners for advice and services for designing core benefits for their workforce. This was often viewed as necessary for recruiting and retaining a high-quality workforce. In an increasingly competitive global economy, these external partners and their services are also critical in order to maintain a competitive advantage.

Table 16. Engagement Levels for External Partners

External Partners	Do Nothing	Level One	Level Two	Champion Company
Health enhancement companies	X	X	X	X
Health plan			X	X
Benefit consultants			X	X
Pharmaceutical companies				X
Primary care physicians				X
Health systems				X
Communities				X
Annual meeting of external partners				X
Effective audit of the external partners				X

"The most effective way to manage change successfully is to create it."
—*Peter Drucker*
1909–2005

Part 2: Transforming Internal Resources

While external partners can be very influential in creating a company's culture of health, the internal environment of the worksite is what employees experience every day. This is what generates their perception of the company culture, and it is essential that they feel this environment supports their well-being. Change in the internal environment most likely is much more difficult than change with the external partners. However, if the vision from the senior strategic leadership (management and labor) is clear, connected to company objectives and shared with all employees, the internal process of injecting health management into the culture might be already done. The environment includes:

1. **Physical environment**
2. **Psychosocial environment**
3. **Human Resource practices, including benefit design**

Environmental-Cultural Assessment

As a first step in the development process, we recommend that both operations leaders and the general employee population complete an environmental assessment of the physical and cultural characteristics of the workplace. The findings will help determine which conditions contribute or do not contribute to a healthy and productive workplace. Since the two assessments are conducted by two levels of the workforce and measure the same aspects of the organization, thus they can be compared to create a "gap analysis." From this analysis, strategies can be formulated to bring the perceived impressions into harmony with the design.

Physical Environment

One of the leading researchers in studying the impact of a health promotion worksite environment is Tom Golaszewski a Professor at the State University of New York at Brockport. He has concluded that, "Focusing on the employee alone doesn't work. We have new theories, new technologies, better trained professionals, and the advantages of outcomes based research. We can deliver slick, individually-tailored and culturally-sensitive educational programs. Much of this has great value. But too often change in our target audience is minimal, short lived or affects a nominal group of employees. In an age of population-based medicine with millions of employees to impact, an exclusive focus on the individual just won't do it. As illogical as it may sound, we may have more success not focusing on individuals, but rather, by primarily focusing on work organizations." Golaszewski describes a health culture as: *A socially and structurally constructed set of core attributes reflecting the prevailing values, underlying assumptions, expectations, and definitions that members of a work organization collectively maintain. The sum of these characteristics affect the way members think, feel, and behave related to matters of personal and group health.*

A company's physical space has often been overlooked in many of early and even current health management initiatives. The obvious environmental targets are vending machines, cafeterias, stairwells, and elevators since nutrition and physical activity are given high visibility in the popular press. For example, what are the options in the vending machines and the cafeterias? Are the stairwells centrally located, and are they dark and gloomy or bright and inviting? Are there non-smoking policies in place? Creating physical space along with organizational policies and procedures that will facilitate healthy behaviors may require many months (or even years) of work.

Onsite fitness centers or memberships in nearby health clubs are popular and often effective; however, a company could consider less expensive options, such as buying each employee a pair of good walking or running shoes—a cost of about $60 a year per person. The walking shoes send the message that one can walk at any time, anywhere. Building or providing memberships at a fitness center might imply that one has to go to a fitness center for physical activity. The extra time that takes could even add to the stress of life. Yet it is well known that physical activity is core to a healthy lifestyle and the presence of an onsite fitness center or memberships to community fitness centers are a very visible sign of the company's commitment to healthy employees. Regardless of how this is addressed, each company should fit the message into their culture.

Some large companies even add medical or health services centers, including pharmacies, to service employees and often even their dependents. The cost of the services is offset by the convenience. At Florida Power & Light, a medical services center is combined with a fitness center to create a fully integrated wellness center.

Psychosocial Environment

"Health promotion has focused on individual improvement, but has yet to fully address cultural influences such as shared values, norms, peer support, cultural touch points and the overall cultural climate. We mistakenly have been trying to get individuals to persevere within nonsupportive peer, household, workplace, and community cultures," states Judd Allen, President of Human Resources Institute. A company's overall culture has to support an emphasis on health and the specific health management program has to be adapted to fit into the culture of the company. The psychosocial environment may be one of the real growth areas in the near future as we learn more about the ways to motivate and reward individuals through the culture of the organization.

Allen defines culture as, "Culture is the sum total of social influences on attitudes and behavior including shared values, norms, peer support, touch points and climate." He then goes on to explain, "Although cultural norms and peer support may be familiar concepts, other cultural elements may be less well known. Shared values are similar to organizational priorities. This concept differs from the more commonly used term personal values. Touch points include such informal and formal influences as rewards, confrontation, modeling, recruitment, selection, orientation, training, relationship development, traditions, rites, rituals, resource commitment, and communication. They are often embedded in policies and procedures. Climate is similar to organizational atmosphere, teamwork, and morale. The three primary climate factors are a sense of community, shared vision, and positive outlook."

"When we empower people to join together in the creation of supportive cultural environments, the influence of social relationships will no longer be viewed as an obstacle to overcome, but rather a virtue to be celebrated."

—*Judd Allen*
President
Human Resources Institute

When the Cleveland Clinic began exploring wellness programming options, physicians there told the planners that they were working at one of the top healthcare facilities in the world, doing interesting and important work, and they knew that meant working a lot of hours. Any wellness program would have to fit into that culture. The physicians said, "Don't tell me to work less, but if you can help me improve my health so that I'm more productive and I can write one more paper this year or see more patients, then I am very happy to work with you," explains Michael P. O'Donnell, PhD, MBA, MPH, Editor-in-Chief and President of the *American Journal of Health Promotion*.

Nurses at the Cleveland Clinic told him: "I am devoted to my profession and I am devoted to my patients. But at the end of the day, I want to go home and have enough energy to be a good parent and a good spouse. And a lot of times, I'm too exhausted. So, help me have more energy and be better able to cope with the stresses of my day so that I can have another life in addition to my work."

Besides meeting employees' goals, participation in wellness programs must also be safe for employees—they have to feel that the time they spend participating does not negatively impact their work or their reputation at work.

Human Resources

Often someone or team of people from human resources is responsible for operations management that drives the whole health management strategy. This is often the best match within the organization since many human resources people feel the responsibility to "grow people" in all dimensions related to their respective needs. The total breath and depth of human resources' responsibilities are beyond the scope of this book. However, it is common for health, benefits, job skills, compensation, motivation, personnel, career paths, recruitment, retention, and other human capital needs to be the responsibility of this unit.

Health cannot be addressed in isolation from all the other factors that make up the profile of a healthy and productive worksite and workforce. "In an increasingly competitive global economy, health promotion professionals need to recognize that productivity happens when people who have the right skills for their job are healthy enough to perform, are well-managed and rewarded for doing great work," says Chuck Reynolds, Principal, Benfield Group. "It makes sense, then, that the corporate executives are focused on the sorts of investments that enable their organizations to attract and keep talented people, manage them well, and pay them for helping to drive business success. No investment in health promotion can make people more productive if they don't have the right skills, are poorly managed or lack incentives to perform; and the investments that are made will fail to engage workers who don't see the connection to their own prosperity. On the other hand, people are more likely to value and protect their health when they see that it enables them to be productive and earn rewards. As such, they can be engaged more efficiently and effectively in programs that will help them achieve better health."

Wendy Lynch, Director of Research at the Health as Human Capital Foundation concurs and states that, "Caring for and about one's health cannot be separated from the context of life and work. A person will value his own human capital (skills, motivation, and health) to the extent that it brings him rewards, enjoyment, satisfaction and/or opportunities. If a company is not prepared to reward high performers well and invest in their skills, efforts to correct health behaviors will likely fall short. Dangling small cash incentives for questionnaires and health programs, in the absence of meaningful bonuses or promising career opportunities, delivers an incongruent message. Either a company values employees or it doesn't; health promotion cannot atone for an environment that stifles overall achievement. Companies have made the mistake of weakening reasons why employees value their health, and then insisting it should matter anyway. We believe significant improvements in employee health will, paradoxically, require redesign of compensation and broad human capital investments rather than more targeted messaging about unhealthy behavior."

Obviously, the success of human resources determines, to a great extent, the employee's perception of the company culture. The following paragraphs touch on some of the efforts of human resources to impact the health and productivity of the workplace and the workforce and the resources should be on the coaches list of resources for referrals.

Career Strategies

Clear career opportunities help give employees the sense that they are on a positive and upward career path; that they are secure and valued in the right company, and want to stay there. Some people view work as an 8 to 5 obligation and view their "life" as being outside of the work setting. They are happy with their family and the balance in their life. Others want to know exactly what they have to do to get to the next level within the organization. Can a workplace meet the needs of these different personal preferences? This is a challenge for the human resource team and options such as work-life balance, job skills, and motivation all contribute to a healthy and productive workplace culture.

Job Design

Job design is critical to the workers' quality of life. American corporations have been pretty good about addressing the physical part of job design, particularly in manufacturing where repetitive motion and safety have been major concerns over the years. Employers are also paying attention to the needs of people who sit in front of a computer most of the day, providing ergonomic devices that improve posture, and reminders to look up every 10 minutes. There is always more to do in the job design area including autonomy around one's work station and efficiency of work flow between employees.

Flexible Working Hours

Flexible working hours where possible, give employees a measure of control over their work life. At the Health Management Research Center, the staff is asked to be in the office between 9 a.m. and 3 p.m. They can distribute another 2.5 hours before or after the core hours. This schedule allows flexibility for attending to child or parent care, taking a class or running errands. We also allow individuals to work from home during times of special need. Obviously not all work environments can offer these options but any adjustments that allow each individual some amount of flexibility can add to job effectiveness and satisfaction.

Benefit design

"Prevention and preventive medicine must be the foundation, not the afterthought, of any effective benefit or an efficient healthcare system. However, because traditionally physicians, health systems, and health plans have not practiced or been reimbursed for behavioral counseling or other clinical preventive services, employers took their lead in benefit design from the experts," states Michael Parkinson, MD, President of the American College of Preventive Medicine. "In the past decade, armed with the convincing evidence of the clinical—and cost—effectiveness of preventive services, employers have demanded, and are seeing differential approaches to the way the providers, benefit plan consultants and health plans approach services that "work" and those that have never been subjected to much scrutiny either at all, or in comparison to preventive care. Consumer-driven health plans with 100 percent coverage of evidence-based preventive care and "value-based benefit designs" reflect the leadership exerted by employers."

Do we continue to select health plans that are the cheapest option and then shift as much cost as possible to employees? Or do we shift toward benefit designs with preventive services and other components that support a health-oriented culture. Forward-thinking employers who are determined to create this culture need to base decisions on quality, not just on cost. For example, generic drugs may or may not be as effective as their counterparts. They represent lower costs, and if lower cost buys the same quality, then that's an absolute winner. But quality over cost deserves consideration in all issues.

Many companies are now considering the amount of employee contributions in relation to compliance and adherence to medical protocol in their benefit design plans. There is concern that if the required employee contribution gets too high, compliance and adherence will most likely fall off. In some cases the lack of prescription fulfillment could result in much more expensive costs in the relatively near future. In this latter case the total costs and medical outcomes both go in the wrong direction.

Individualized benefit designs would allow employees to choose high deductibles or low deductibles based on their approaching medical needs. With flexibility in place, an employee may plan for that knee or hip operation and perhaps lose a few pounds in preparation for the rehabilitation process. In fact, sometimes the weight loss makes the hip or knee operation unnecessary. Another critical aspect of benefit design is enabling individuals to choose the best physicians and health systems to maintain or improve their health status.

Healthcare initiatives are part of the trend toward consumerism: teaching and motivating individuals to be self-leaders. Organizations can support this process through the use of incentives, transparent actions, and an emphasis on improved and maintained health status

Incentives must follow an actionable behavior. The long-standing entitlement mentality associated with insurance really does not encourage individuals or organizations to grow and learn. (Incentives are discussed in detail in Chapter 10.) Benefit consultants and health plans can provide valuable information and experience in providing information about new incentive programs that work. It is often the case that incentives other than financial work well in promoting the desired behavior. This is a critical area for the company to get correct as health management is moved into the core culture of the company.

Incentives Must Follow Actionable Items.

Transparency means access to information that enables people to find the best doctors, the best hospitals, and the best medications. To achieve transparency, employers must provide employees with data and then help them interpret it in terms of costs and quality. Health plans have the opportunity to offer additional value to employers and the members they cover since they have the quality and cost data. They can share information that illustrates gaps in physician care and infection rates for hospitals, two routine measures of quality. Because employers will still be paying for sickness care, finding the best, most cost-effective physicians and healthcare systems are in everybody's best interest. In addition benefit plans can be designed, in cooperation with the health plan to ensure that employees and dependents have open access to the best physicians and other health professionals, in terms of quality services and costs. Another factor that should be considered is ensuring unlimited time for employees to have access with healthcare professionals.

Health status, the major emphasis in our health management strategy can be impacted by benefit design, and health status is the single major emphasis of this book. How do employees and their families develop and maintain the highest health status possible? In our opinion, high health status is the ultimate goal in healthcare. In fact, regardless of which health plan is offered now or in the future, individuals and organizations always win when people are in optimal health.

"Our goal is to use the insights gained from identifying health risks to implement action plans that result in employees reducing their risks. Specifically, while striking a balance between personal and corporate responsibility, we strive to offer health care benefit plans that encourage individuals to take responsibility for choices that are known to adversely impact their health, while acknowledging the need for some structure through integrated health care that maintains and improves healthy lifestyles."

—*Joel Bender, MD, PhD*
Corporate Medical Director
General Motors

Consumer-driven (high-deductible) health plans are gaining popularity and could be a valuable tool in helping employees become self-leaders and taking responsibility for their own health. But to be successful, employers must do their part by designing the plans carefully, adequately funding them, and educating employees in their use. Health status becomes even more important to employees who learn that they are spending their own money for their healthcare. However many people could have a tendency to avoid or postpone medical visits; which emphasizing the importance of preventive healthcare is a key part of the education process.

Another innovation that we would like to see is a move to coordinating benefit design and integrating with program design. Often these design decisions have been made in isolation from one another. As a result, a design feature or access to coverage in one area could impact another area. For example, changes in disability coverage could impact medical/pharmacy expenditures or vice versa. Behavioral health, employee assistance programs and pharmacy are often separate sections of a health benefit plan requiring separate plan designs. This is counterproductive. The solution is to involve all the stakeholders in creating effective and value-based benefit designs. In addition, most often the company will sponsor programs and the design of these programs should meet the needs of the benefit designs. For example, programs could be designed to help employees get the most quality out of their medical, disability or financial benefits. "It's essential for us to have population health management and benefit design as an integrated approach," says Wayne Burton, MD, Medical Executive at JP Morgan Chase. "In order for us, the country, to better manage healthcare costs trends and population health, it needs to be an integral part of our benefit plans and benefit plan strategy."

The strategies described above can help employers recruit and retain their top employees. In the magazine industry, where a high turnover rate for editorial employees is common, Rodale's mission to support the health and well-being of staff members has had a positive effect. People join the company and are amazed by the scope of the programs that we offer—which other publishing firms are not providing, "says Amy Plasha, Vice President of Compensation and Benefits.

How It Works

In working with the employer members of the Midwest Business Group on Health, President and CEO Larry S. Boress has found that to keep health benefit costs low, employers need an "extreme makeover" in their own "House of Benefits." "The foundation for this new 'house' must be built, based on knowing the covered population's needs, maintaining a healthy workforce—one that is capable and motivated to stay healthy, using cost-effective providers and drugs and reduce the risk of disease in partnership with vendors who understand the employer's expectations for the entire covered population."

Steve Barger and Michael Wilson, former President and Executive Director, respectively, of the International Foundation of Employee Benefit Plans, have some very insightful thoughts around the future structure of benefit plans if they are to become more impactful to employees. "Over the last several years strides have been made in getting employees, employers, board members of trust funds, unions, and providers to understand the intrinsic value of the health of the workforce and U.S. population in general. During this time the focus has been mostly on disease management, preventative measures and incremental system changes. Employers, trust funds, payers, and providers have developed several 'schemes' to address cost, efficacy, and efficiency. And although some progress has been made to date, these efforts and the acceptance of these efforts have been far short of expectations for improvement of overall health status for individuals or creating a positive impact on access, quality or the cost of healthcare in the U.S."

"Because of the convergence of a number of factors, i.e., change in political leadership, significant societal desire to see improvement in the current system, innovative programs focused on health and quality of life (rather than disease management and prevention), and the current financial crisis that confronts the U.S. and global economy, the time for changing the U.S. healthcare system is now. There has never been a clearer mandate to move ahead on both structural system changes and benefit plans that truly focus on the achievement and maintaining of health and quality of life factors. It will take the diligent pursuit of both structural and benefit plan design change initiatives to achieve a successful redesign of the U.S. healthcare. One without the other will not be affective in achieving desired results in quality, access, cost, improved health and enhanced overall quality of life for the U.S. population."

"Integrated multi-modal programming, significant linkages to benefit incentives, personalized and targeted communications and strong cultural norms for wellness will be necessary to move the wellness agenda forward in the American workplace. The vitality of our efforts along with our persistence in pursuing this vision will ultimately determine the outcome. This is neither an easy challenge or one that we can ignore."

—Larry Chapman, MPH
Senior Vice President and Director of the WellCert Program
WebMD Health Services

Summary and Engagement Scoring

The areas of opportunity discussed in this section are core to the environment or even the culture of the company and thus what each employee experiences during each workday.

Table 17. **Engagement Levels for Internal Partners**

Culture Considerations	Do Nothing	Level One	Level Two	Champion Company
1. Environment				
a. Ergonomic evaluations	X	X	X	X
b. Food services for choices		X	X	X
c. Vending machines/food services/etc.		X	X	X
d. No-smoking policies		X	X	X
e. Flexible working hours			X	X
f. Job design				X
g. Stairwells configured to encourage use				X
h. Clinic/wellness center				X
2. All procedures aligned with healthy culture				X
3. Clear career paths				X
4. Benefit Design				
a. Acute care covered	X	X	X	X
b. Condition (disease) management		X	X	X
c. Employee Assistance Program (EAP)		X	X	X
d. Health benefits focused on quality outcomes				X
e. Shift from entitlement to consumer mindset				X
f. Transparency for services				X
g. Health status				X
5. Spouse and dependent eligibility			X	X
6. Corporate Survey for Culture of Health				X
7. Employee Survey for Culture of Health				X

Part 3. Implementing the Health Management Program

Are You Ready to Implement?

Operations leaders should not rush the move to Pillar 3 (self-leadership) until the majority, if not all, of the above partners demonstrate commitment—and that is not likely to happen within the first six months, to a full year. The internal partners' buy-in is especially important. At minimum, policies and procedures must be aligned with the vision for a healthy and productive organization. It is important that the employee see and experience the company's commitment to a healthy and productive culture in alignment with the vision created by the senior strategic leadership (management and labor).

Once those criteria are met, companies can proceed toward implementation for the mid-level and first line leaders (managers) and eventually the population of employees, possibly including a timeline for engagement of spouses and other dependents.

The Next Step Toward Self-Leader Implementation

So in summary, senior strategic leaders create the vision, conceptualize the business case for health management within the company and in a series of meetings, the senior leaders share these objectives with the operations leaders who incorporate their own perspective. Commitment from the operations leaders is critical, because they create the environmental and cultural attributes that are needed to support the vision.

Concurrent with mid-level planning, companies will find it advantageous to form a health management committee of influential employees who are willing to be part of the design process. Clearly, union representatives should be involved in creating the vision and in the early program design stages as well. By creating opportunities for employees at all levels to be engaged in the planning process, companies are also fostering the supportive environment that is critical to culture change.

Barger and Wilson write that, "To make a difference in the workforce, we must focus on improved quality of life while engaging the interest of employees, employers, trust funds, unions, and providers. When we connect this interest with the positive impact of an improved quality of life on productivity and healthcare expenditures we will have success.

"To achieve success, we must communicate with our employers and employees in a manner that will engage them in managing their healthcare. We must have buy in from corporate officers, plan sponsors, workers and their families. This can only be achieved by involving all effected parties from the get go. Too many times well intentioned programs are presented to workers without involving the participant or worker in their development and then we wonder why we have such poor utilization.

"For our purposes, success is defined as a healthy and productive population that grows the economy providing an improved quality of life for all citizens."

Final Step Prior to Implementation

Implementation is best accomplished by first managing expectations of the individuals at all levels within the organization. Understanding the vision, the benefits to the company, the benefits to the individual, and the components of the program and the expectations of them becoming their own self-leader is critical prior to any roll-out. This is best accomplished by a series of meetings with all levels of leadership (company and union), followed by small group meetings with the rest of the total population. Everyone has to understand the vision of a healthy and productive company and the benefits to each (company, managers, union, and all individuals). Finally in those small group meetings the details of the cultural enhancements and of the health management program should be explained in terms of what will be expected of each person as they continue to develop as a self-leader.

"C-suite support is necessary but not sufficient for success. Equally or more important is having grass-roots level support for the programs. If results are not achieved, the C-suite will lose interest and withdraw support over time. As a result, program leaders need to 'sell' the concept not just to the C-suite, but to the 'masses' (e.g., individuals, families, sites) as well."

—*Cathy Baase, MD*
Global Medical Director
The Dow Chemical Company

Summary and Engagement Scoring

The success of the implementation totally determines the success of the total cultural implementation. The process of engaging each of the external partners, the enhancement and integration of all of the internal resources, and the mobilization and engagement of all of the managers and of the total population will ensure success in moving toward a culture of health.

Table 18. **Engagement Levels for Implementation**

Implementation Considerations	Do Nothing	Level One	Level Two	Champion Company
1. Senior Leadership Support			X	X
2. Senior Leadership Vision				X
3. Commitment and Integrated use of External Vendors			X	X
4. Commitment and Integrated use of Internal Partners				X
5. Use of Internal Resources		X	X	X
6. Integration of Internal Resources				X
7. Commitment of Leaders at all Levels				X
8. Discussion of Expectations for all Employees				X
9. Transparency of Objectives at all Levels				X
10. Programs designed to find gaps in resources				X

Final Word

"The stars are all aligned. You have the health plans saying this is the right thing to do. You have benefits people hearing it. You have the senior executives at the corporations saying this is what we have to do to manage our healthcare costs and that it is the right thing to do for employees.
This is a golden window of opportunity for our country."

—*Wayne Burton, MD*
Medical Executive
JPMorgan Chase

Chapter 10: *Self-Leadership Creates Winners*

Third Fundamental Pillar to Support the Health Management Strategy

"Every human being is the author of his own health or disease."
—*Buddha*

Population Self-leadership—from the Grass Roots up

The third pillar of the overall health management strategy is the population. With public health being a notable exception, America has always focused on the individual whether in sickness care, disease prevention or health promotion. In addition, each of these services has adopted the medical model: wait for sickness, then treat with pharmaceuticals or surgical solutions; or, detect high risk, then treat with risk-reduction strategies. Even preventive services are focused on early detection of disease or risk for disease.

This chapter is divided into two sections: Part 1 focuses on ways to provide individuals with opportunities to take an active role in becoming self-leaders in their health status and overall well-being. Part 2 focuses on encouraging participation within the total population. Incentives are a part of the motivation and they will be discussed in Chapter 11.

Obviously, no one wants to be sick. The real question is, do you want to be healthy? Do you want to move beyond "absence of sickness" to high-level wellness? No program can bestow wellness. People have to assume self-leadership for their health, and then companies can provide resources to help them recognize and address any risk factors that may be discovered.

As a first step in achieving this mindset, individuals should have the opportunity to complete a health risk appraisal questionnaire and participate in screenings and health counseling. Then, they need to contact a health coach, who can help them think through their individual situations and point them to the right resources based on their health status and objectives. Finally, they should have the opportunity to participate in at least two wellness activities or programs throughout the year. These could be individual or population-based programs Individual-based programs could be related to risk reduction, general nutrition, well-being, or physical activity. Population-based wellness programs are an integral part of the optimal health-oriented culture and environment: they could include general weight maintenance, know your numbers, or general walking programs. Everyone is eligible to participate and everyone can be a winner.

Part 1. Driven by Individuals in the Population

Individuals do best if they understand that health is vitality and energy, not just the absence of disease, and that they are their own self-leaders in charge of improving or maintaining their own health status and influencing the health status of their families.

Health Risk Appraisal: Questionnaire and Profile

The health risk appraisal (HRA) system is core technology to integrate health into the culture of a company. The system begins with a HRA questionnaire, which can be customized to the person, company or location and delivered in paper or web formats. Some companies are more interested in specific health-related risks or behaviors than others. For example, a trucking company, concerned about its drivers making long hauls, might want to ask additional questions about sleep patterns, while a manufacturing company may be more concerned about joint flexibility in relation to musculoskeletal injuries. After completing the questionnaire, each employee receives an individualized profile calculating his or her risks and health status. These profiles can to be customized or tailored to the characteristics of the individual, for example, by age, gender, risk levels, and number of preventive services undertaken. There is a wide range of HRAs being used; some are simply risk calculators, others are health education tools, still others actually calculate risks for disease morbidity or mortality, and finally the HMRC includes a calculation related to expected cost within the next two to three years. Some HRAs are a combination of the above.

Biometric Screening

The second part of the HRA system is biometric screening. These screenings are provided by local health professionals, by focused screening companies, or by health enhancement companies. Perhaps the most important component is that after the screening, a health professional spends time with the individual reviewing the results. The purpose of the screening is to determine the blood levels of the several components of cholesterol (HDL, LDL, and total cholesterol), glucose, and triglycerides, as well as blood pressure, waist size, body weight, and height.

"People have to know their cholesterol levels in order to change them," says Alberto M. Colombi, MD, MPH, Corporate Medical Director at PPG Industries, where more than 75 percent of the company's 33,000 employees have taken an HRA and understand where they stand on the healthcare continuum. "Our employees have been exposed to the concept that risks drive diseases and that they have a correlating cost," Colombi says. "We tell them that in order to affect healthcare costs, we have to manage health. If we manage health, we may finally affect productivity and costs at the same time. That means we have to prevent anything that is preventable."

"This is a societal problem. The demands placed on the healthcare system are going to be almost overwhelming in the next 30 to 50 years, but healthy eating, exercise and the end of tobacco use could decrease the demand for medical services by a remarkable percentage."

—Paul Handel, MD
Senior Vice President and Chief Medical Officer
Health Care Service Corporation

These screening sessions can be expanded to include dental, hearing, vision, flexibility, strength, bone density, and other services that are generally included in an annual physical exam in a physician's office. In many cases, the counseling session also covers the HRA profile if it is printed at the site. Thus, the individual completes the HRA questionnaire, has the screening, and immediately receives a counseling session and HRA profile. People highly value this procedure. One of the limitations is that this very information-dense session may deliver too much data for some people to comprehend all at one time.

Some managers are reluctant to allow an employee to take 30 to 60 minutes to complete this activity. This becomes an issue of values, but also may indicate that the operations leaders need to more fully convince the mid-level managers of the company's commitment and expectations to bringing about a culture of health.

Health Coach

The third component of the HRA system requires the individual to contact a health coach. Everyone can use a coach! If you are at low risk, you need a coach to help you find the resources to retain your champion status. If you are at high risk, a coach can help you address your risk factors or refer you to resources within the company or community. If you are coping with a chronic illness or disease, a coach can help you stay on your prescribed regimen or refer you to an appropriate disease management or behavioral health specialist. Coaches are often available as part of the health plan's total health program, through a health enhancement company's HRA system, or provided by the company as part of its health management program. Any of these plans might also include access to private coaching specialists.

"When you treat an individual, you are not just treating one disease or one problem. You are treating the whole individual. So if I am obese, it's not just the obesity you're treating. You may also be treating diabetes, hypertension, heart disease and depression. So benefits have to provide resources to treat the whole person. That's the way you have to look at it."

—*Andrew Scibelli*
Manager of Employee Health & Well-Being
Florida Power & Light Company

Typically the coaches will have access to the HRA and screening data when the participants contact them. The data are made available in a variety of formats, from a simple list of the risk factors, to a list of the participants' responses to all the questions on the HRA, to a sophisticated prioritization of the risks and other analytical analyses. Often the data available to the coach is a combination of the above. The HMRC uses a trend management system which uses the dangerous risk combinations, prioritized risk, clusters, rank order, and recommended level of intervention to inform the coach of the relative importance to the person's future cost or disease.

As a health enhancement company working with Crown Equipment Corporation and other employers, Achieva Lifetime Health learned what individuals need and want from employer-based health coaching programs. Janet Walker, a company co-founder, found that everyone in a population, regardless of risk level, benefits from one-on-one contact with a health coach as part of follow-up programming. By integrating health coaching with the completion of a health assessment, companies set the stage for a higher annual level (over 90 percent) of participation in the coaching process and for a higher level of motivation," she suggests. "They begin to see that they are in control of their health and that they can make positive decisions that lead to positive actions."

The goal of the coaching sessions, as well as the total goal of the Health Management program is to develop self-leaders, regardless of health status. The coach can help individuals identify their strengths and their weaknesses and learn to utilize those strengths (time, energy, resources, friends, etc.) to create and maintain a healthy and productive environment and lifestyle. In addition, the coach can help clients learn to cope with their weaknesses so they do not remain barriers.

"A health advisor who can help individuals understand their HRA results and assist them in making decisions is the most important tool we have for getting people engaged."

—*James R. Heap, MD*
Medical Director
Crown Equipment Corporation

Amy Schultz, Director of Prevention and Community Health at Allegiance Health, tells us, "Our coaches' goal is to have an engaging, motivational conversation around healthy behaviors. We don't say, 'You ought to change.' Instead, we ask, 'What would make you want to change?' or 'What makes you want to stay healthy?' That's different for every person, and when someone has that 'a-ha' moment, it is very powerful."

Cindy Bjorkquist, Director of Wellness and Care Management Consulting, Blue Cross Blue Shield of Michigan agrees. "You have to really unlock the story of each individual, and the way to do that is through individual coaching. Every person has a story. People don't want to be overweight. They don't want to be sedentary or in pre-disease states. But there are so many factors as to why people have these difficulties. You have to figure out what their fears are, what their needs are, and help them to change their lifestyle and build their new story."

"We're seeing a realization that boots-on-the-ground, face-to-face interactions can be very cost effective, and can improve participation and program outcomes. It's very powerful when practitioners are 'coaching by wandering around,' as opposed to expecting employees to come to them. A 'Point of Service' coaching option provides greater opportunities for 'brushes and touches' that reinforces the wellness brand and reinforces the health culture."

—*George Pfeiffer, MSE*
President
The WorkCare Group, Inc.

With coaching strategies and appropriate incentives in place, we find that over 90 percent of the eligible individuals participate in the total HRA System, which begins to define "engagement." Participation that leads to engagement by 85 to 95 percent of the population is the major positive outcome from coaching. In some organizations, the current but ineffective practice is that a health coach calls only the high-risk HRA participants. This ends up involving less than 20 percent of the participants, and only 5 percent are still participating after one year.

The data in **Figure 28** (on page 136) show the results of this type of coaching model. No system can make a difference in an organization with such low participation and a focus on only the high-risk individuals. Over a one-year period, as the process proceeds from the total number of HRA participants all the way to the number of participants who are still engaged after one year, the percent of the population continues to decrease. At the end of the first year less than 2 percent of the population was participating in the coaching program even when the original identification indicated that 24 percent of the population was at high-risk and thus eligible for coaching. We refer to these data as our "step-down" or "waterfall" results.

To reverse these disappointing results, we recommend that everyone, regardless of health status, must contact a coach; this is integral to the program's success. The bars in **Figure 29** (on page 137) compare results between the "coach will call you," with the step-down results with "you contact the coach," which brings higher results. The strategies at the bottom of the graph increase the engagement rate and the results now approach a rectangular engagement pattern. At the end of the first twelve months the cumulative participation rate should be approximately 70 to 90 percent.

The difference between the "coach will call you" and the "you contact a coach" models is the difference between 10 percent and 80 percent participation in the coaching element of the HRA System.

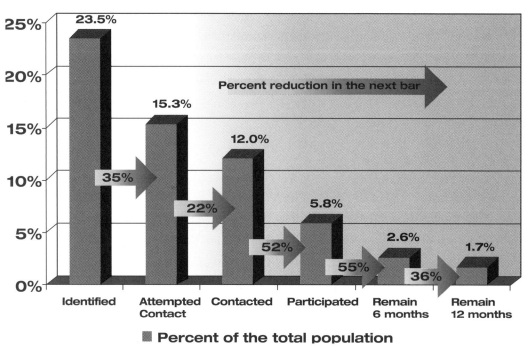

Figure 28. **Observed Program Attrition Rates**

Lynch, Chen, Edington. JOEM. 48:447-454, 2006

Both employees and spouses can be and should be included in this strategy if an organization truly wants to make a difference in the total population.

"We see the best results when an employee and a spouse are trying to make changes together."
—*Karen O'Flaherty*
HealthWise Manager
Crown Equipment Corporation

The coaching strategy incorporates an active referral program. Coaches don't need to solve problems. They help people become self-leaders so they can solve problems independently. The most effective coaches consider the whole person and not just the risk or the disease. They avoid "telling"

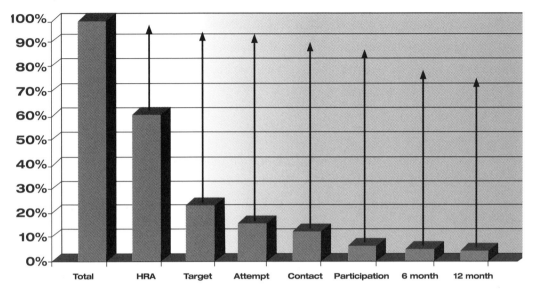

Figure 29. **Intervention: High-Risk Strategy**

- Vision from leadership, preparation (why, what, purpose) for a health risk appraisal (HRA)
- High premium reimbursement, better plan,...
- Everyone contact a coach
- Coaching style and content for everyone
- Unlimited contacts (inbound/outbound)

Target: rectangular engagement pattern

individuals what to do, guiding them instead to solve their own issues. Margaret Moore, President and CEO of Wellcoaches and a pioneer in the coaching field, observes, "The humanists taught us that homo sapiens are wired to self-actualize, to be happy and healthy, and that certain conditions are needed to enable us to be our best: our relationships and our environment. Therapists, and now professional coaches, have shown us the power of close growth-promoting relationships (personal or group) that combine empathy and affirmation with a courageous call to rise above challenges and grow."

In the process of developing a self-leader the coach could begin by working though the participants' perceived barriers, and then transitioning to their strengths and finally to helping them chart a course of action. If the individual is still struggling or the problem warrants it, the coach may then suggest solutions or other resources, such as a physical fitness program, a behavioral health program or a condition management team. Even if the individual is referred to a specialist, the coach remains the primary contact.

The coach should never forget job related skills and motivation resources that may be available to the employee. Often a poor skill set related to their job demands could be the source of poor performance and could lead to health risks or health problems.

Likewise it seems as though most employees run into motivational issues at one time or another. Even a referral by the coach to Spencer Johnson's book, *Peaks and Valleys,* could be enough to provide some early skills around life management.

"Our best organizations have shown the power of corporate culture and cultural permission to improve population-wide health and happiness. The time is now to bring to bring masterful coaching to organizations to accomplish both—growth-promoting relationships and cultures."

—*Margaret Moore*
President and CEO
Wellcoaches, Inc.

Earlier coaching models provided three or six contacts. Our recommended coaching component has no limits or time table although in terms of keeping people engaged, a minimum of two contacts are recommended. One should occur soon after the health assessment, and one during the fourth quarter of the program year. The rationale for this recommendation is to maintain engagement throughout the year. The company is sending the message that employees have unlimited resources available to them: "You do what you need to do, and we'll stay there with you: this benefit is not going to expire."

It's interesting to note that even with unlimited contacts available, the number of contacts is three. Some individuals contact the coach only once, while others need as many as 20 contacts.

Unlimited commitment by the company is the right message. Just as the company undertakes finding the best doctors and the best health systems to take care of its people when they get sick, it pledges unlimited resources to help its people stay well.

"Our health coaches run programs for low-risk people. We absolutely believe the healthy group needs guidance and help to stay healthy as well."

—*Michael L. Taylor, MD, FACP*
Medical Director for Health Promotion
Caterpillar, Inc.

Web-Based Interventions

In addition to onsite and telephone interventions, there has been a major increase in internet use. Web-based interventions are relatively inexpensive and available to anyone with access to the internet. The interventions could draw upon pre-programmed curriculum or be highly interactive. The potential of this intervention media is still being developed but some of the initial programs show promise. Healthmedia, located in Ann Arbor and recently acquired by Johnson and Johnson, continues to be a leader in Web-based tailored programming. Vic Strecher, University of Michigan professor and founder of Healthmedia, created a sustainable solution by providing multiple ways to tailor the right message to each individual's learning style. He states, "It's quite clear to nearly everyone that our lifestyles and behaviors have a deep influence on our health status. This influence is increasingly being quantified and used in predictive modeling of healthcare costs and productivity. The real challenge in my opinion is to move upstream and change the behaviors that increase healthcare costs and reduce productivity. The science of health-related behavior change has matured to the point that we're now able to tailor behavior change programs to very specific psychosocial and behavioral factors at an individual level. With the emergence of interactive communications technologies, like the Internet, we can now tailor effective behavior change and disease management programs to literally millions of individuals at a low cost."

Wellness Programs

The final component to this individual-based health management strategy requires each person to participate in at least two wellness programs throughout the year in addition to coaching. These could be programs recommended by the coach, by the HRA or by some of the general population-based programs described in Table 20 (on page 144) of this chapter. The purpose here is to maintain engagement throughout the year.

The desired outcome from this individual-focused strategy is to create self-leaders who engage in their own decision making. Self-leadership is critically important for the sustainability of any program, especially the aspect of maintaining a high-level (low-risk) health status. Why? Because we know that when left alone, the natural flow of individuals is to a higher risk status.

"We need to get as much of the total population engaged and participating in health initiatives as possible. It's not like the old legacy aspects of disease management where we were focusing on the 10 to 15 percent of the population that were driving 80 to 85 percent of the annual medical and pharmacy claims costs. That's good, but it's not sufficient. We have to move upstream and also help the other 85 percent of the population focus on their health so that they don't develop those chronic conditions."

—Ron Loeppke, MD, MPH, FACOEM, FACPM
Executive Vice President, Health and Productivity
Alere

Summary and Rating the Individual-Focused Programs

Individual and single-focused programs, most often aimed at risk reduction, are still the basis of many wellness programs.. These programs, however, miss the opportunity to get individuals engaged in a holistic way and keep the low-risk people at low risk. We now know that everyone needs to participate in the full HRA System of questionnaire, screening/counseling, coaching, and two or three other programs to achieve success.

Table 19. **Engagement Levels for Individual-Based Programs**

Individual-Based Programs	Do Nothing	Level One	Level Two	Champion Company
Health Risk Appraisal				
Standard HRA with risk prevalence/generic profile		X	X	X
Risk prevalence/tailored response/tailored resources		X	X	X
Prioritized risks and preventive services				X
Screening				
With BP/weight/cholesterol/HDL		X	X	X
With BP/weight/cholesterol/HDL/waist/glucose/other			X	X
With mental health/environmental assessment				X
Counseling				
Comprehensive counseling post HRA and screening		X	X	X
Counselor to refer to other resources				X
Coaching/Advocate				
Coaching for high risk and condition management		X	X	X
Coaching using predictive modeling for individuals				X
Coaching for all people				X
Health advocate coaching utilizing referral				X
Wellness Modules				
Health communications		X	X	X
High-risk reduction programs		X	X	X
Low-risk maintenance programs				X

Part 2. Population-Based Programs: Built into the Culture

"We can be best in class at addressing acute and chronic illnesses, but that will only be 25 to 30 percent of a company's employees in a given year. It's being able to have an equally positive effect on the quality of life and the vitality of the other 70 percent of the population that will have the biggest impact."

—David Cordani
President and COO
CIGNA Corporation

From the strategy of providing HRAs, screening, coaching on a one-one-one basis, and individual-based programs, we now move to programs that engage with the company's total population. This is the second key component of integrating health into the culture of the company. Total population programs help the low-risk people stay low risk, encourage all employees to develop a winning attitude, nurture the champions and begin to engage those higher risk individuals in the culture of health.

For example, one program where everyone can win was illustrated in Table 1 (on page 31). Over a six-month period, participants set out to walk 500 steps a day, learn their numbers (blood pressure and cholesterol), and maintain their body weight. Everyone has the incentive, and because everyone can do these three things, the organization can now celebrate its winners. OK, what's next? The next step might be to ask the individuals what they would like to undertake for the next six months: perhaps 1,000 steps, still don't gain weight, or still just know their numbers, And, off we go for the next six months of the journey to better health.

The destination of the journey is determined by each individual when he or she arrives at a personal sustainable level of these three health-related factors. Other "one step at a time" programs could be devised for most of the risk and lifestyle factors related to the health and productivity areas.

"One may walk over the highest mountain one step at a time."
—John Wanamaker
Philadelphia businessman, 1838–1922

Think about it. You're "not going to getting worse." You're eating healthier and taking the stairs because you want to maintain your weight. No pressure to do more. Hey, you did it this month. You still weigh the same. You didn't gain weight. You can do it. Maybe next month you'll try to lose a pound or two – or maybe not. If after another month or two you are at the same weight—you are still winning.

Building winners, one step at a time. The first step? Don't get worse.

A health-oriented environment reinforces the population-based strategy. Eliminate the signs by the elevator that say "take the stairs, it is good for your heart" and replace them with signs that say "take the stairs and get a prize," such as a pack of sugarless gum or an apple. Perhaps people will walk up the stairs to see the prizes. As part of a "take the stairs" program, make those stairs inviting: safety, music, carpet, good lighting, handrails, and prizes at key locations.

Another key part of a population-based health management strategy is to engage everyone in skill development and motivational opportunities. A highly productive employee is not only healthy but one that also has competitive skills for the requirements of the job and is highly motivated to be a champion within the champion company. Coaches can also be facilitators by directing individuals to resources to meet these needs.

> *"If you can maintain risk status over a two-year period, that's a huge success."*
> —Renae Sieling
> Health Educator
> Wisconsin Education Association Trust

In addition to the "don't get worse" challenge, more traditional risk-reduction programs are needed for those who decide, in consultation with their coach or through their own initiative, that they want to undertake a more intense self-improvement. Thus companies should provide wellness programs for individuals who are determined to lose weight, quit smoking, manage stress, etc. These programs should be covered by benefit plans, but only at the point when individuals enroll and attend the programs. Table 20 (on page 144) presents a sample menu of behavior change programs.

Table 20. **Population-Based Resources**

■ Weight management	■ Business specific modules
■ Physical activity	■ Career development
■ Stress management	■ Communications
■ Safety belt use	■ Financial management
■ Smoking cessation	■ Social/Information networks
■ Nutrition education	■ Clinic or medical center
■ Disease management	■ Ergonomics
■ Online information	■ Vision
■ Nurse line	■ Dental
■ Newsletters	■ Hearing
■ Behavioral health & EAP	■ Chiropractic
■ Pharmacy management	■ Complementary care
■ Case management	■ Integrative medicine
■ Absence management	■ Physical therapy
■ Disability management	

"Our employee wellness initiative is going great. We have a whole suite of programs in place. The culture has changed, and people are excited about it."

—Paula M. Sauer
Vice President of Care Management
Medical Mutual of Ohio

In 2004, the Centers for Disease Control and Prevention sponsored a project at the California Department of Health Services (DHS) in Sacramento with the intention to study the impact of changes in the environment on health status and productivity measures. Over a three-year period, the DHS implemented 13 health interventions and environmental changes including organizing a farmers market within walking distance of the office buildings. They sponsored "take the stairs," "know your numbers," and encouraged healthier food choices at a nearby deli.

At the end of three years, although no individual behavioral change programs were implemented, the health risk status of the overall population improved dramatically. The group not only beat the natural flow of risks but emerged with higher aggregate health status. In addition, overall absence rates declined. The results clearly verify that creative, health-promoting procedures, policies, and programs can have powerful results.

"Creating an evidence-based program to keep employees healthy is a worthy undertaking for any employer, public or private."

—Sandra Shewry
Director
California Department of Health Services

As President of The Wellness Council of America, a national not-for-profit business and health organization with a rich history in workplace wellness, David Hunnicutt has witnessed, "…a renaissance of sorts in the last several years. Employers of all shapes and sizes are embracing health management concepts in a way that hasn't been seen since the safety and industrial hygiene movement took hold early in the last century. Because of the strong link between lifestyle, medical costs, and organizational productivity, employers are embracing population health management concepts with zeal. And, in my mind at least, this alone is reason enough to be optimistic about the future—even in the midst of economically challenging times.

"When American Business gets engaged, things change.

"As we move forward with our quest to link health and well-being to bottom-line organizational outcomes, it is imperative that we remember that corporate health management initiatives are something we do with and for our people—not something we do to them.

"In an age when CEO's salaries are 400 times that of the average worker (as compared to 40 times in 1970), we must remember that by many economist's accounts, the typical worker is making less now than they were in 1970. As a result, many employees are highly skeptical of employer-led health interventions."

"As we leverage more than two decades worth of research and strive toward 'zero trends,' it is my belief, that to be successful, we must strive to engage the U.S. workforce in a partnership whereby employers and employees alike race to find common ground in promoting good health at the worksite."

"As a result, health will become a shared priority and our field's efforts will be indelibly integrated into the very fabric of the organization's culture"

—David Hunnicutt
President
Wellness Councils of America

Summary and Ratings for the Population-Based Programs

The objectives of population-based programs are maximum engagement and a design that ensures everyone can "win" by participating. The majority should be able to reach the intended goals over a designated time period.

Table 21. Engagement Levels for Population-Based Programs

Population-Based Programs	Do Nothing	Level One	Level Two	Champion Company
Communications		X	X	X
Population programs based upon achieving outcomes		X	X	X
Programs offered by Web, Onsite, Offsite				X
Population programs based upon everyone winning				X
Pedometers at 500 steps per day				X
No weight gain				X
Know your numbers				X
Training programs: people, communications, supervisor				X

Building a Program at PPG

PPG decided to begin at "the base of the iceberg," Alberto Colombi says. More than 25,000 people, or 75 percent of the company's 33,000 employees, have now taken a health risk assessment and understand where they stand on the healthcare continuum.

To help support employees and change the firm's risk profile, PPG has set up a network of 71 wellness teams throughout its worksites. Factory workers, union representatives, engineers, and secretaries are all participating in the wellness movement.

While wellness programs have typically been small in scale and in scope, PPG takes a broad view of its health management programming and sees it as part of an overall effort to control healthcare costs and remain competitive. Components of the plan include:

1. Prevention. PPG is educating employees and providing programs to modify behaviors and address healthcare risk factors such as smoking and lack of exercise.

2. Preventive services. The firm is encouraging employees to take advantage of preventive services covered by health plans, such as mammograms and flu shots.

3. Benefit design. PPG is asking employees take more responsibility for their healthcare costs by paying a greater share.

4. Challenging waste in the healthcare system. As employees take on more responsibility for their own health in terms of risk factors and cost sharing, PPG is striving to educate them on how the healthcare delivery system works, how they can avoid unnecessary use of services, and how they can get the most out of services they do use.

"The underlying goals of wellness are becoming part of the company's culture," Colombi says, "and that will lead to real change."

Final Word

"Employers excel at solving problems and turning them into opportunities. That is what business exists to do. So businesses have to stay in the health arena. These are population-based problems, and businesses are very good at creating systems and managing populations."

—Sean Sullivan
President and CEO
Institute of Health and Productivity Management

Chapter 11. *Reward Positive Behaviors*

Fourth Fundamental Pillar to Support the Health Management Strategy

"As a society, we have spent years punishing people for bad health behavior, but we have never really rewarded people for good health choices."

—Mike Huckabee
Former Governor of Arkansas

Positive Reinforcement Is Key to Success

Most of human nature runs on positive reinforcement and reward, and so it is natural for organizations to create incentives to motivate and reward members of the workforce. Incentives come in all shapes and sizes, although cash rarely fails. One can usually predict an increase in participation as the incentives become more meaningful to participants, from a low of 10 percent for no incentive to a high of 100 percent when the incentive is coverage by the company's health plan. In addition to the initial incentive, smaller rewards prove necessary throughout the year to create and maintain engagement.

Incentives and positive reinforcement are an important component of both individual- and population-based strategies and probably represent the tipping point for generating effective engagement. Everyone knows that behavior change is not easy, and perhaps not even possible without special circumstances. It is clear that people benefit from additional resources in their efforts to achieve and maintain low risk. Pharmaceutical agents, for example, can provide a critical component of the intervention to help with risk reduction programs such as blood pressure, glucose and cholesterol control. Drugs can also be useful in behavioral change programs such as smoking cessation, weight loss, stress or anxiety management, and depression management.

Often, people don't think they need to change because they have not confronted a crisis. They are not sick or bedridden or hospitalized. By yesterday's standards of thinking, they are healthy, not realizing that real health represents a higher level of vitality and energy. So Americans and others throughout the world have been slow to embrace wellness programs, and companies have been slow to integrate health into their corporate culture as a serious business and economic strategy. We now know that our expectations have to change if we expect to live a low-risk lifestyle throughout our lives.

The way to survive is to bring incentives and corporate reinforcement and rewards into the picture. Sure, there will always be those who say, "What do I have to do to get the incentive, just find a coach? OK, I'll make that first contact." Actually, it is that simple. Once an employee makes the contact, it becomes the coach's role to help individuals appreciate the total value of health for themselves, their families, the company, and the community, and to challenge those persons to become self-leaders.

Initial Incentives

Companies should share their mission with employees—"Your health status impacts you and our company—that's why we are undertaking this program." Typically the initial and major incentive is tied to benefits: perhaps as much as 20 percent of the cost of individual health coverage. Most incentives need to be at least in the $600 to $1,000 range to convince at least 90 percent of employees to participate. In addition to cash or premium reduction, some companies offer the incentive of a more generous health plan or the option of a health savings account.

"We give people incentives to take a health risk appraisal and to follow up. They get a $200 reduction in their health plan premium. You also have to pay $50 per month more if you're a smoker. It's an integrated approach. The opportunity to save money on healthcare gives people an incentive to join our wellness program, which has a 75 percent participation rate."

—William B. Bunn, III, MD, JD, MPH
Vice President–Health, Safety, Security and Productivity
Navistar, Inc.

Many companies have reached the point, and we endorse this strategy, of recognizing health status is too important to be tied only to benefits. These companies have made a step to make health management a core business strategy. One consequence of this move is that if an employee engages in the health management strategy such as the health risk appraisal system described in Chapter 9, the company will pay for his or her healthcare. Employees who decide not to participate will pay for their own healthcare benefits.

This is an example of a successful business reward program that often results in 100 percent initial participation. Whatever the strategy, it should be discussed openly during the preprogram meetings with the operations leadership and employees as a way to attempt to manage expectations.

Table 22 shows several levels of incentives with the corresponding expected levels of participation. A company should determine its desired level of participation and then be prepared to provide the corresponding level of rewards or incentives.

Table 22. Influence of Incentives on Initial Participation

Incentive	Participation
■ No incentive	2%–10%
■ Passive incentive	15%–25%
■ Small item incentive	20%–35%
■ Cash incentive	20%–40%
■ Benefit plan improvement	30%–60%
■ Benefit plan plus cost reduction	50%–70%
■ Combination of benefits and cash	75%–100%

Follow-up Rewards for Positive Actions

Once motivated by the initial incentive, participants need another series of rewards to maintain their interest and engagement. A sampling of such rewards is shown in Table 23. This second level of positive rewards (incentives) is necessary because the initial activity probably occurs at the point of benefit selection and then is likely forgotten until next year. The emphasis on a healthy lifestyle must continue throughout the year in order to reach the desired outcome, a culture of health.

For example, if you go to a nutrition seminar, you get a hat. If you go to another "lunch and learn," you get a T-shirt or you get $25 applied to your debit card. Other incentive designs allow you to accumulate points which can be exchanged for products, trips or cash. Constant communication keeps the momentum going and keeps participants engaged, either maintaining their health status or making improvements.

Table 23. Positive Reinforcement

- Culture reminders (managers, leaders)
- Cash, debit cards ($25 to $200)
- Benefit design (HSA contributions)
- Hats and T-shirts
- Population programs
- Surprise events
- Decorate stairwells
- Special cafeteria/vending offerings
- Organizational rewards (departments)

"The good thing about health promotion is that people generally see the benefits right away. They feel better, so that eventually becomes the intrinsic incentive."

—*Michael P. O'Donnell, PhD, MBA, MPH*
Editor-in-Chief and President
American Journal of Health Promotion

Another effective incentive technique is to have the activities of the current year lead to a qualification threshold for the maximum benefit plan or further incentives for the following year. Regardless of the size or type of incentives used, it is clear that they must not be viewed as entitlements: that is, effective incentives must follow actionable behaviors.

In some cases, a negative incentive might prove effective, such as charging additional dollars for smokers. Non-participants in the health management program might be told that they will not qualify for the enhanced or standard healthcare benefit, but be relegated to the most basic plan. All levels of leadership (senior, operations, and self-leaders) will form a powerful and influential force in designing these various positive reinforcements, and are critical to keeping the company and its members moving in a positive direction.

Incentives Follow Actionable Behaviors.

Many health management programs are conducted for members scattered throughout a broad geographical region. More than 100,000 teachers and pubic school employees in Wisconsin count on the Wisconsin Education Association (WEA) Trust to provide insurance plans that help them and their families become well when someone is sick and, increasingly, help their families stay well when they are healthy. What's most important is that Al Jacobs, former President and CEO of the Trust, created an environment that supports and celebrates wellness. It offers health education consultants to the school districts, a health risk appraisal that clearly demonstrates to employees what their risk factors are, it offers telephone support and coaches to individuals who need help achieving their goals, and it recognizes and rewards healthcare champions—those who are healthy and those who have worked to improve. People with good cholesterol numbers receive congratulatory letters and are offered services to help them maintain their health, similar to the services offered to those who want and need to get better. Like many firms already embracing health management ideals, WEA Trust's next hurdle is to substantially increase participation from 60 percent to 90 percent. When nearly all of its members take advantage of its wellness programs, Jacobs believes WEA Trust can reduce healthcare costs by as much as 25 percent.

"Jobs in the public schools can't be outsourced overseas. We have to get this right."

—*Al Jacobs*

Past President and CEO

Wisconsin Education Association Trust

Summary and Rating the Effectiveness of Rewards for Positive Actions

Companies utilize rewards to recognize positive actions, and most organizations use incentives to motivate and reward individual members of the workforce. Incentives and rewards should be used to sustain positive behaviors and to maintain engagement throughout the year.

Table 24. Engagement Levels for Incentive and Positive Rewards Programs

Incentives Programs	Do Nothing	Level One	Level Two	Champion Company
No Incentives	X			
Passive incentives (T-shirts, hats, gym bags)	X	X		X
Small item incentives (book, pedometer)	X	X		X
Cash or premium reduction		$25–$100	$250–$600	$600–$1,500
Hats and T-Shirts throughout the year			X	X
Rewards earned for prizes throughout the year			X	X
Premium benefit plan			X	X
Benefit plan plus education in contribution				X
Cash or debit cards throughout the year				X
Engagement, company pays; no engagement, employee pays				X

Final Word

"Help people reach their full potential. Catch them doing something right."

—*Ken Blanchard, Spencer Johnson*

The One Minute Manager

Chapter 12: *Quality Assurance: Outcomes to Drive Success*

Fifth Fundamental Pillar to Support the Health Management Strategy

"Health management programs today have to be data-driven and evidence-based. You have to have data to understand what the problems are in your population, and you have to use science to develop the right kinds of programs to attack those problems."

—*Michael L. Taylor, MD, FACP*
Medical Director
Health Promotion, Caterpillar

Quality Assurance: Measures Provide for Continuous Improvement

Evidence-based outcomes measures are the hallmark of a successful health management strategy. The results of the program offered and the effects of changes in the environment have to be fed back into the process for continuous quality improvement.

First, the company has to demonstrate a high level of "organizational engagement" by committing to the five fundamental pillars of the health management strategy. Achieving the full benefits of the culture of health means that the company is commitment at level four: a champion company.

Second, companies must demonstrate a high level of "employee or member engagement" as assessed by,(1) percent of individuals actively engaged, with a goal of 85 percent to 95 percent, and (2) percent of employees at low-risk status, with a goal of 70 percent to 85 percent of the total workforce. Additional financial metrics would be specific to each company but would include costs (medical and pharmacy) and time away from work (absenteeism or presenteeism) per employee or per covered life. Additional metrics would include appropriate employee satisfaction measures, follow-up culture/environment assessments, specific program evaluations and other measures that provide valuable input into quality assurance leading to effective decision support.

"We have seen good results from our wellness program and safety initiatives, including a 10 percent reduction in lifestyle-related healthcare claims."

—*Dick Davidson*
President, CEO and Chairman
Union Pacific Corporation

Data, Information, Knowledge, and Decision Support

Nearly all companies, small to jumbo, have access to data so data availability by itself does not seem to be the critical or limiting factor in quality assurance. A sampling of the data that could be available for companies is shown in Table 25.

For a basis level of decision support it is not necessary to capture all of the suggested data unless the company wants to dig deeply into the analytics. Much of the data that are needed for quality assurance can be gathered from participation and engagement rates, employee satisfaction and overall healthcare and productivity trends.

Table 25. Datasets Needed to Get to the Total Value of Health to an Organization

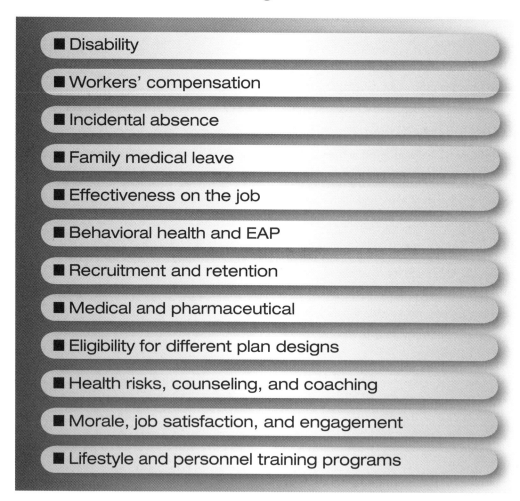

- Disability
- Workers' compensation
- Incidental absence
- Family medical leave
- Effectiveness on the job
- Behavioral health and EAP
- Recruitment and retention
- Medical and pharmaceutical
- Eligibility for different plan designs
- Health risks, counseling, and coaching
- Morale, job satisfaction, and engagement
- Lifestyle and personnel training programs

The data identified in Table 25 are also the bases of an advanced assessment of quality assurance. The flow of this journey is shown in Table 26. The final step is sometimes the hardest since the individuals reviewing the information have to have a detailed working knowledge of the purpose of the health management investment and of the overall vision, goals and objectives of the senior leaders That is, from the company's point of view the real value comes in the last step: "How can all of this knowledge be used to provide support for decision making, such as investments in training, benefits, environment, work schedules, and other critical contributors to the health and productivity of the workplace and workforce?"

Table 26. Quality Assurance

- Data feeds come from all possible sources (warehouse)
  - Create benchmarks within each data set
  - Integrate data into a datamart
  - Create integration between data sets

- Information is discover from examining the associations between all data elements
  - Access plan design to create synergy between data sets
  - Study the relationships between health, disability and productivity

- Knowledge comes when relationships are connected to outcomes critical to company strategy and vision

- Decision support points Integrate the knowledge to create the accessible and effective

Driven by Success: Efforts Aligned with a Healthy Workforce

Decision support is a critical component of integrating health into the culture of the company. In the past, efforts to assess the economic value of wellness programming primarily focused on the return-on-investment (ROI). While much of the discussion in this book has been around economic outcomes, there are other equally and possibly even more important outcomes—the information that gets produced and fed back into the system for continuous quality improvement. Measuring the results of health management efforts provides quality assurance and decision support so that the programs can be continuously evaluated and then enhanced.

Companies should be asking, "How do we keep improving the workplace and how are our efforts aligned with supporting a healthy and productive workforce?" That's where quality improvement programs make a difference: How are you doing and how are you meeting your quality goals? Stakeholders will want to see that investing in a healthy culture is adding value to the organization.

Saving money is an exceedingly important outcome measure, but it is only the result of high-quality, effective programs for the total population.

Assuming a company implements the five pillars of a health management program, operations leaders will have developed a scorecard that not only tracks progress on their total quality management criteria but also supplies information on business and economic objectives of the company. That is, are the results consistent with the objectives defined in the vision statement developed by senior leadership? Achieving the criteria for a champion company will bring the company to a fully functional, comprehensive, and sustainable health management program.

Proof of Concept

When organizations find solutions to perplexing problems, sometimes it is difficult to know how, where or to what extent various strategies contributed to that success. When success happens, all hands go up to claim credit. In the case of health management, the answer lies in the data. Participation and engagement rates, health risks, and cost analyses will show the extent to which improvement in health status led to improved health and productivity outcomes.

Five Necessary and Sufficient Components of the Proof of Concept

1. Demonstrate that the change in the percent of low risk for the two-time HRA participants beats the natural flow of risks. This demonstration is valid only if the engagement rate is high (somewhere above 90 percent of the total eligible).

2. Demonstrate that the change in the percent of low cost for the two-time HRA participants beats the natural flow of costs. As above, this demonstration is valid only if the engagement rate is somewhere above 90 percent of the total eligible.

3. Demonstrate that the change in the percent of low-cost individuals for the total population beats the natural flow of risks and costs.

4. Demonstrate that the annual cost trends for the company show a lower rate of increase over the previous several years; a lower trend rate than that of benchmark companies; and, eventually, a trend rate that approaches zero or negative trend.

5. Demonstrate that the total savings exceeds the total cost of the program or at least that the savings equals the cost. Total savings should consider recruitment and retention of high-quality employees and contribute to corporate community responsibilities.

Note. It should be obvious from the above set of measures that obtaining a very high participation rate is essential in order to prove the total value of the health management strategy. The high level of engagement is necessary to overcome the "participation bias" often seen in these types of calculations. That is, a group of two-time HRA participants who represent a small fraction of the workforce is clearly a biased sample and should probably be dismissed as such. In that case, positive results, including high ROI values, are highly unlikely to make a difference in the organization.

The only way to obtain credible data is to get to a high engagement rate within the total population, measure all the outcomes, and calculate the results in the terms that make a difference in the organization. Expressing savings in terms of shareholder value, number of branch offices operational, number of work-years added, or any other business terms commonly held as a measure of company success is absolutely essential.

"More than 95 percent of the employees who receive benefits through our company are enrolled in our wellness program, and there's a pervasive recognition that the health of our employees is as important as anything else we do here. You can have a great program, but if you are not impacting the majority of people, you haven't achieved a culture change."

—Amy Schultz, MD, MPH
Director of Prevention and Community Health
Allegiance Health

Summary and Scoring of Measurement

Measurement for quality assurance, continuous improvement, evaluation and decision support, and economic outcomes are all crucial and absolutely central to the success of the health management strategy. In addition to the metrics listed here and throughout this book, there are other specific data that can be tracked to facilitate a smoothly running program, such as engagement by specific units or populations, outcomes from specific initiatives, participant response to specific programs, and many more options. Table 27 on page 161 summarizes measurement by levels of engagement.

Successful Outcomes (Scorecard)

There are a variety of economic, social, physiological, sickness, wellness, and other measures that can be used as a scorecard to chart a company's progress in moving toward a culture of health. However, the vast majority are influenced in one way or another from two fundamental metrics:

1. **Percent of the population engaged in the health status strategy**
2. **Percent of the total population at low-risk health status (0-2 risks)**

**Table 27. Measurement, Evaluation, and Decision
Support by Level of Engagement**

Measures	Do Nothing	Level One	Level Two	Champion Company
Employee satisfaction		X	X	X
Employee participation		X	X	X
Scorecard (percent participation)		X	X	X
Reduction in health risks		X	X	X
Return on investment		X	X	X
Decisions based upon program results			X	X
Employee engagement				X
Scorecard (percent engagement)				X
Scorecard (percent low risk)				X
Total value of health (sum of all outcome measures)				X
Proof of concept (beat natural flow)				X
Proof of concept (bend the trend lines)				X
Company specific economic indicators				X

"One of the keys to being a good leader is having an end in mind or purpose, commonly referred to as the 'vision thing,'" says Bill Greer, Head of Benefits for Kellogg Company. "Everyday when I come into work, I remind my team that our group's mission is to improve the 'health and wealth' of Kellogg employees. Although health and wealth are related, our biggest focus has been on improving the health of Kellogg employees and their dependents. That's a lot easier when you have metrics. Our key metric, working with the University of Michigan Health Management Research Center, is to improve the percent of our population that is low risk (two or fewer risks). We have been successful in increasing that percentage from 55 percent in 2005 to 65 percent in 2007 with an overall goal of 70 percent to 80 percent of our population low risk.

"And the most important part—our executives are convinced that improving the health of our employee population as measured by this simple metric will lead to improved business results via lower healthcare costs, improved productivity and higher levels of engagement. Having said that, our biggest challenge going forward is figuring out which parts of our Feeling Great programs (exercise, weight loss, flu shots, coaching, etc.) have the biggest impact on health risks. That will be a critical step for us if we are to meet our goal of having 70 to 80 percent of our population low risk."

Once an organization accumulates sufficient data, the economics of even a mere 1 percent change in the percent of the engaged population can be calculated. The same type of calculation can put a dollar value on the change in the percent of the total population at low-risk health status. These calculated outcomes can be used to estimate or model future enhancements and accurately assess the total value of health to the organization.

Measuring the economic value of health should be given at least equal priority to other measurement analyses in the organization.

"We are seeing much more rigor around how these programs are structured and less fluff kinds of activities. There is also a bigger burden on all of us who are in this industry to have data showing that we are making a difference."

—Michael L. Taylor, MD, F.A.C.P.
Medical Director for Health Promotion
Caterpillar, Inc.

Net Cost per Participating Employee. Tom Welsh has spent much of his thirty five years in business in the finance field including serving as the CFO at Pittsburgh Plate and Glass (PPG). PPG, being a manufacturing company, needs to be keenly aware of costs and margins. There is a relentless pursuit of more effective/efficient manufacturing methods and a very high degree of scrutiny over investments which drive cost reduction, increase value and provide sustainable advantage. A good idea, which is not thoroughly supported with the proper homework on the numbers, is likely to be dead on arrival.

Due to the environment at PPG, it was critical to pose the health initiative in the same framework as other initiatives that were competing for resources. "As such," says Welsh, "We applied an identical measurement and justification process to the health initiative as we would for any manufacturing investment process. We identified, mutually agreed to pertinent cost metrics, and then measured and communicated them in a framework which was clear, consistent, and in conformity with manufacturing reporting. Through this approach, we were very effective in getting the attention of management at all levels.

"We did this through year over year comparison of understood and clear metrics valued against reliable benchmarks. We developed scorecards which compared internal facilities on an apples to apples basis and we clearly demonstrated the value generated from attention to health."

One good example is illustrated in Figure 30. We educated employees and management on the metric of net cost per participating employee. "Our population is actually a good bit older than the benchmark and therefore we would be doing well to just be maintaining our year over year increase at the benchmark level. We are still finalizing the accounting for 2008, but for the duration of our metrics, we believe we can confidently say we have saved $114 million as a result of being better than trend. This is a visible overall metric, but is supported by similar financial metrics, charts and report cards that go down all the way to the plant level and in some cases even more granular. These measures help reflect the outcome of the numerous health awareness, health cost mitigation, and behavioral changes that are initiated and executed at each operation. The reporting helps keep a continuous cycle of innovation and attention to health cost and therefore health."

Figure 30. **Net Active Healthcare Cost**

Percent Change Per Participating Employee

Cumulative Savings 2002 to 2007 = $114 million

Benchmark / PPG

Year	Benchmark	PPG
2001	12.1	9.2
2002	11.5	7.4
2003	10.2	5.8
2004	9.0	4.9
2005	6.7	-2.5
2006	6.1	5.1
2007	6.0	8.2
2008	6.3	3.4

Data to end of Q3 2008 (12 month RA)

Benchmark source: Mercer

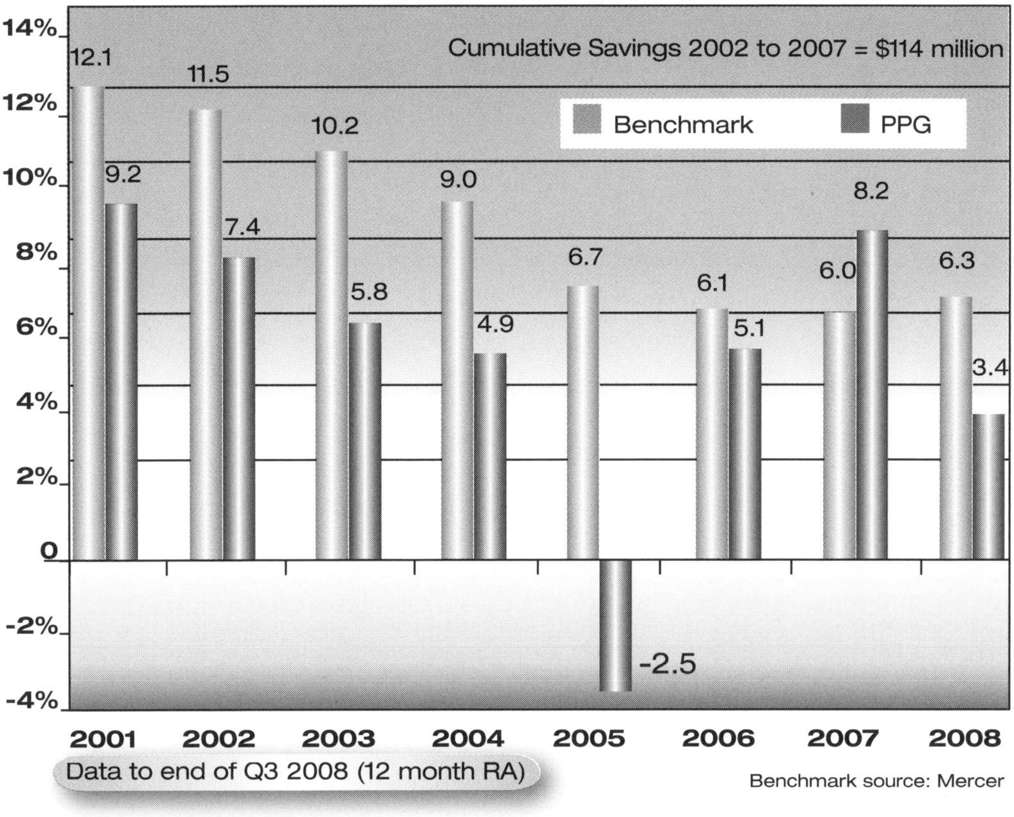

Total cost of employee health. Dublin is a municipality in which employees have enjoyed a historically rich medical plan. Like all employers who provide medical benefits to employees and families of employees, the City of Dublin was aware that the double-digit increases in the cost of providing those benefits could not be sustained indefinitely; nor does it reflect good stewardship of public dollars. David Harding, Director of Human Resources, and co-workers Mary Kay Ruwette, Human Resource Manager, and Michelle Hoyle, Budget Manager, determined after a thorough review of their program that, "… the 'consequence of doing nothing' would result in an increase in claims costs from 2005-2008 of nearly 47 percent over three years. Although our original wellness efforts focused on reducing the rate of the growth in the costs of our benefits program, we realized quickly that the long-term key to managing the costs of providing healthcare to employees and families was to reduce the preventable risks in our population. Based on the theory that cost follows risk, we believed that engaging employees in managing individual risks would in turn control the City's costs. So far, the theory has worked in practice—we have been able to maintain a more modest rate of claims cost increase of closer to 5.5 percent per year.

"What began as a City Council directive to explore cost-sharing with employees has evolved into a comprehensive health management effort—Healthy by Choice. One way to measure the impact of Healthy by Choice is to measure the 'total cost of employee health'—a measure that includes claims as well as absenteeism and workers compensation costs. In 2006, it was estimated that our total cost of health per employee would increase to $12,184 for 2009. Based on actual data through 2007, the projection for 2009 now has been revised downward to $9,899 per employee, or a decrease of nearly 19 percent.

"What sets Dublin apart is the public sector environment—each step of Healthy by Choice has been discussed in a public forum and reviewed and blessed by an elected body, the Dublin City Council. The Dublin City Council showed foresight and faith in the inception of this program—in looking beyond the immediate 'fix' of cost-shifting to employees, and faith that a more strategic and long term approach would work."

"With health promotion and prevention, it always ultimately requires effective engagement. Health promotion is not something that you do 'to' people or 'for' people but is rather done 'with' people. The integrity of the program and the people build trust. Delivering something of genuine value sustains engagement. I am absolutely convinced that achieving significant outcomes is possible."

—*Cathy Baase, MD*
Global Medical Director
The Dow Chemical Company

Summary and Scoring for Program Engagement

Table 28. Estimated Outcomes* for the Different Levels of Program Engagement

The outcomes are directly related to the company engagement level.

Outcome Measures	Do Nothing**	Level One	Level Two	Champion Company
Percent participation (Cumulative over three years)		40%	60%	90%-100%
Percent engagement ***(Cumulative over three years)		20%	40%	85%-95%
Percent low-risk		50%-60%	60%-65%	75%-85%
Cost of program per eligible employee per year*		$75	$150	$400
Savings over first three-years per eligible*		$50	$50	$800
Savings in the fourth-year per eligible*		$100	$400	$1,600
The Annual Report contains an explanation of efforts to integrate health into the culture of the company				X

*Costs and savings are dependent upon inflation rates, initial risk, cost situation, and company
*Costs and savings are only for medical plus pharmacy benefits; additional savings will result from calculations of time away from work and presenteeism.
*Turnover rate is not included in these calculations
**The Do-Nothing and Early-Transition Levels are built on real data from the HMRC
**The Champion Company level is the result of our simulation based upon the results from our Corporate Consortium members.
***Health Risk Appraisal plus three or more coaching sessions plus two other participations

Case Study of an Emerging Champion Company

One Midwestern manufacturing company launched its efforts to become a Champion Company in 2004 and has remained committed to that strategy. Its engagement rate has been over 90 percent in each of the program years (HRA, screening, coaching, and one other wellness program where available). The data in **Figure 31** show how the total employee population increased in medical and pharmacy costs from 2002 through 2007 (the latest data available at the printing of this book). At the time the program was implemented, the population could be stratified by both cluster membership and prioritized risk levels, then their respective costs were followed from 2004 through 2007. The data clearly show the expected increases, with the low-risk individuals being and staying low-cost; the medium-risk individuals increasing in costs at approximately the same rate as the total population; and the high-risk individuals increasing at a much higher rate. There appears to be a moderation in costs during the latest year, which could be attributed to the changes in the workplace culture or changes in benefit design. The key point illustrated in **Figure 31** is that there is a separation of costs over time related to risk levels.

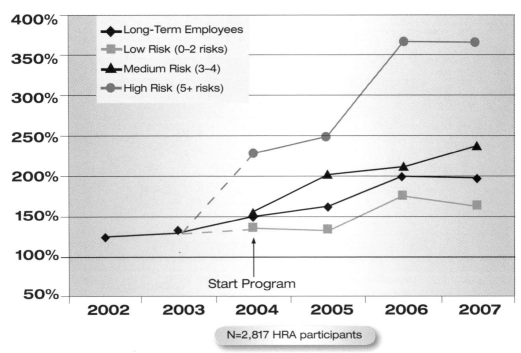

Figure 31. **Average Annual Contract Cost of Long-Term Employees Split by Relative Health Risks After the Start of the Program**

N=2,817 HRA participants

A second analysis examined the same individuals from 2004–2007 (see Figure 32), looking at changes in risk levels. This allowed for four years of the program to make an impact. The summary of the Markov Chain for risk analysis shown in Table 29 (on page 168) shows that the risk changes clearly beat the natural flow changes of the "do nothing trend." The natural flow would predict that the percent of low risk would decrease by four to six percentage points and the percent of individuals staying low risk would be approximately 78 percent. At this company the percent of low risk individuals increased by 11 percentage points and the percent of those staying at low risk over these three years was 81.

The Markov Chain for 2006–2007 costs showed positive results in that the company beat the expected natural flow. The company showed a one year increase in those at low-cost (plus 3 percent) and with 86 percent of the low-cost individuals staying low-cost. We did not introduce the natural flow of costs in this book although it was mentioned in the proof of concept criteria. The natural flow of costs would estimate that a population would lose up to 2.5 percent of its low-cost population and approximately 74 percent of the population would stay low-cost over two years. Clearly this company beat the natural flow of risks and costs.

Figure 32. Risk Transitions Over Time

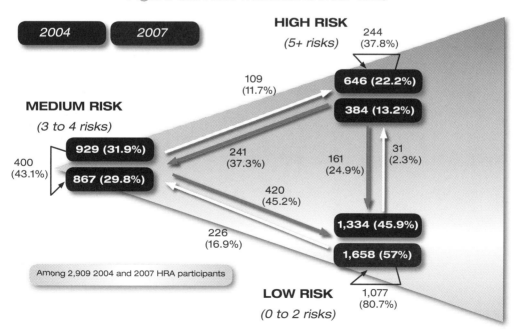

This manufacturing company is approaching meeting all of our proof-of-concept and Champion Company criteria by not only changing health but changing cost outcomes for specific individuals and the population as a whole.

Table 29. **Risk Transitions Between 2004 and 2007**

	Do Nothing Trend	**Actual Change**
Change in Low-Risk Status	Decrease 4 to 6 percentage points	Increase 11 percentage points
Percent of Low Risk Remaining at Low-Risk Status	75%	81%

Conclusion

It is finally clear that after all these years, we now know how to design a health status strategy that can be integrated into the culture of the company. It makes serious business and economic sense, benefiting organizations and individuals. We know how to design and implement steps to engage all levels of leadership. And finally, we now know how to measure the total value of health, to the company and its workforce.

Final Word

"This book is a road map for tackling some very big issues—healthcare costs and abundant living."
—Margie Blanchard, PhD
Co-Founder and Former President and CEO
The Ken Blanchard Companies

Going Forward

"We must become the change we want to see in the world"
—*Mahatma Gandhi*

Chapter 13. *Implications for Public Policy*

"You don't have to see the whole staircase, just take the first step."
—*Martin Luther King, Jr.*

What Is the Connection to Public Policy?

Corporations are often the ones footing the cost of sickness. That is the reason why 30 years ago we at the Health Management Research Center chose to work exclusively with businesses. Corporations are best positioned within society to make a commitment to maintain a healthy and productive workplace and workforce because they get the immediate return.

My feeling is that health policy is too important to be left to medical or public health officials, especially based on the results we have seen over the past many decades. It seems like business leaders would be better trained to engage the whole population and impact the total value of health for our nation.

"Employers are agents of change. Even more government-oriented policy thinkers—those who think it's the government's job to act as a regulator—believe that large employers play a key role in fostering innovation at a speed unimaginable by government agencies. Employers can also fine tune, pilot, and test out ideas quickly so that we can all learn. We need that nimbleness and flexibility to learn what programs and policies work best."

—*Helen Darling*
President
National Business Group on Health

Regardless of who leads the decisions around health policy, access and affordable healthcare are the right things to do on the sickness side of the health-continuum. However, equally important is that worksite and population-based cultures and overall health status are the right things to do on the wellness side of the health-continuum.

As we watch the most committed and engaged companies achieve success through promoting changes in the workplace culture and the health status of the workforce, individual employees, and their family members face the challenge of maintaining their healthy changes in communities that fostered unhealthy behaviors. Helen Darling observes, "The unraveling of the financial system has demonstrated that the private and public sectors are more intertwined than ever before. Employers—private and public—are able to reach and support their employees and dependents on an ongoing basis. Their policies and programs have a tremendous impact on their populations. Since these policies and programs affect more than two-thirds of the people under age 65, what they do or don't do has significant public policy implications." Once again, it is clear that ultimate behavior change must engage the workplace environment, neighborhoods, communities, and all segments of society. Public policy changes must occur to allow this change to take place.

"Worksite wellness needs to be recognized as a much more strategic activity for global employers. The potential of the workplace as an environment for the efficient and effective management of the health of a population needs high level policy recognition and support. The alignment of individual, organizational, and societal objectives in shaping the health of defined populations represents one of the most important policy challenges of the 21st century."

—Larry Chapman, MPH
Senior Vice President and Director of the WellCert Program
WebMD Health Services

Premises

1. Health is too important to leave to the medical profession and their sole focus on sickness care. America has one of the best sickness care systems in the world and we will continue to need its resources to care for the sick. Health is too important to leave to public policy specialists and politicians and their emphasis on access and "affordability" for sickness care. Access and paying for sickness are extremely important issues that need to be addressed, but they will not solve the quality and economic issues of the continually escalating healthcare crisis.

2. No amount of money that we throw toward the problem will be sufficient to provide for sickness care and accommodate the decreasing productivity of our citizens if we continue to accept the "natural flow" toward increasing health risks, disease, and costs. It is too late when our current approach is to essentially ignore the most healthy of our citizens, wait for sickness, and then attempt to fix the problems. This strategy has been proven to be linked to unmanageable increasing costs and of questionable quality.

3. When we consider the total value of health to the total population, total health management is the only solution that touches each and every individual in the country. It is also a win-win for everyone because it results in reduced pain and suffering in individuals, decreasing cost of sickness for our corporations, and an increase in productivity and prosperity for our corporations, families, communities, states, and country.

The problem we have before us is unsolvable at the level of thinking that got us into this healthcare crisis. It is clear that more doctors, more nurses, more hospitals and more traditional medical research are NOT at the level of thinking that will get us out of this healthcare crisis.

Although access to care and affordable healthcare are the right things to do, they too will NOT get us out of this healthcare crisis.

The only solution is to elevate wellness care to the same priority level of sickness care and thus enter into a higher level of thinking that WILL get us out of these healthcare and productivity crises!

Action Items

A wide variety of public policies must be developed to

fix the systems that lead to the defects.

Individuals alone cannot solve the healthcare crises; corporations alone cannot solve it; communities and states alone cannot solve it, and neither can the federal government. This calls for a coordinated effort on behalf of every element of society.

Worldwide, people realize that philosophically we need a new way to do health management. The solution also needs to focus on fixing the societal systems that lead to the defects. Just as we improved worker safety and addressed the issues related to the quality of our products, we can solve the healthcare crisis.

No one is as smart as all of us.

It is well beyond the scope of this book to suggest detailed policies for all levels of society; however, we know that it will take a national cooperative and synergistic effort for America to be successful. It is clear that there are a whole host of potential players in this endeavor. Each has its own self-serving objectives, which have been evident for decades. Below is a sampling of the players (stakeholders) and their goals. Working together, we can all make a difference in the way we tackle health (sickness and wellness) in America and:

- Individuals: stop getting worse as the first step to winning
- Corporations: implement the five fundamental pillars of the health management strategy
- Communities: form coalitions of stakeholders to create community cultures of health
- State Governments: fund state and local strategies to implement cultures of health
- Federal Government: fund strategies to impact total population health, including sickness and wellness.

Final Word

Our premise is that the Five Fundamental Pillars of the Health Management strategy can succeed not only for companies but communities, states, and the country.

Chapter 14: *Final Words*

"Never doubt that a small group of thoughtful, committed citizens can change the world. Indeed, it is the only thing that ever has."

—*Margaret Mead*
1901–1978

Challenge to Businesses

The business case we presented in the introduction and first six chapters is real and well documented in our work and the work of many others. The solution we presented in Chapters Seven through Twelve is a challenge to companies to "raise the bar" in terms of commitment AND engagement. We know of no company that has reached the destination but we acknowledge many who are well into the journey and who have served as pathfinders in working toward a champion company.

Realistic Challenge for Implementation

We do not expect any company to adopt the five fundamental pillars and completely implement them in a totally linear and chronological fashion. We believe in small wins and just don't get worse as the first step, even for company strategy. However, the vision, commitment, and engagement of the leadership must come first followed by a visible first step in creating a healthy and productive environment/culture. After these steps the journey has begun with a total implementation timeline of perhaps two to three years, or longer in some cases.

Review of Ten Simple Concepts

1. Companies have proven that the "do nothing" or "wait for sickness" strategy is unsustainable.

2. Companies need to change their definition of health from "absence of disease" to "high-level vitality," and approach health as a combination of sickness and wellness strategies.

3. The business case for health management indicates that the critical strategy is to "help the low-risk people stay low risk." Or as we like to put it: "help the healthy people stay healthy."

4. The first step is "don't get worse." Let's create winners, one step at a time.

5. Effective healthcare strategies must target the total population of an organization in order to capture the total value of health to individuals and to the organization.

6. The challenge for organizations is to "create the vision, create the culture, market, execute, measure, and make it sustainable."

7. Companies need to engage "partners, not vendors." This includes the health plans, benefit consultants, primary care physicians, pharmaceutical and health enhancement companies and eventually health systems and communities.

8. An effective overall strategy starts with a clear vision from the leadership that is consistent with corporate objectives followed by engagement of all of the internal partners in creating a company culture aligned with the healthy and productive vision.

9. Companies need to get to "full engagement of the leadership and of the total workforce" in order to bend the trend lines and get to "zero trend" in each of the outcome measures.

10. "Clear vision from the leadership," translates to adopting the Five Fundamental Pillars of Health Management to build a corporate culture of health and to grow into a healthy and productive workplace and workforce.

University of Michigan Health Management Research Center Commitment

We will continue to "grow the learning tree" (see Figure 22 on page 71) in partnership with our Corporate Consortium and other organizations. Our primary focus will remain in the science of health (wellness and sickness) as a business or economic strategy. There is much work to do and new frontiers to challenge us. We welcome partners in this journey.

What's the Point?

One of the questions I ask at the end of nearly every presentation is, "What's the point?" Why do we do this? I don't know the answer, I just raise the question! Of course I know it's about health, and of course it's about economics. But to me, it's really about people helping people. How do we help each other? How do we help each other get through this life with a minimum amount of pain and suffering? It's not about disease or risk factors or money. Of course it is. But the overriding purpose is how do we help each other avoid pain and suffering? How do we create healthy families and healthy companies where we work and healthy communities were we live? How do we live lives full of vitality and energy with a high level of well-being? This is a serious challenge for America, our citizens and for every country worldwide, companies and people. I don't know of any group of people in the world who does not support a passion for this mission.

"It is health that is real wealth and not pieces of gold and silver."
—*Mahatma Gandhi*

Our Sense of Passion

I hope we have conveyed our sense of passion and urgency for organizations and individuals to find a new way to do health management in this country and worldwide. We can no longer wait for people to get sick, no matter how much it is in our tradition to take care of the sick. We cannot watch people become high risk, although it may be possible to recover some of those risks. We cannot allow champion, low-risk individuals to drift toward medium- and high-risk and then to disease and high-cost. We must create a total health management strategy by adding wellness strategies to the existing sickness strategies. We must not only help individuals to manage their diseases and to reduce their health risks but, more importantly, we must help these self-leaders not get worse. There is little time left in terms of business survival. We must all feel and act on the urgency to move this to center stage on the health agenda.

Final Word

> *"We live very close together. So, our prime purpose in this life is to help others.*
> *And if you can't help them, at least don't hurt them."*
>
> —Dalai Lama

Let's help each other avoid unnecessary pain and suffering.

Let's not get worse, as the first step in getting better.

Let's help those who do get sick, not get any worse.

Let's help each other stay as healthy as possible.

Let's help the healthy people stay healthy.

Quotes from Leading by Example. Partnership for Prevention 2005, 2007

Partnership for Prevention® highlights employee health management programs. Leading by Example: Leading Practices for Employee Health Management. Copyright © Partnership for Prevention® 2005 and 2007. The full publications may be downloaded free of charge on Partnerships Web site, www.prevent.org/LBE. The quotes were excerpted from the publications with permission from Partnership for Prevention® based on the 2005 and 2007 publications.

2005

2007

112 Readings

56 Selected Publications from the HMRC: Corporate Consortium Members
(Chronological Order)

1. Garman, J. Fred, Jesse A. Berlin, Dee W. Edington, Linda K. Curtis. Towards a Healthier Organization. *Current Municipal Problems.* 9:141-145, 1982.

2. Edington, Dee W., Louis Yen. Worksite Health Promotion Utilizing Health Risk Appraisals. *Proceedings of the Society of Prospective Medicine.* 21:37-39, 1985.

3. Pfeiffer, George, Dee W. Edington. Health Risk and Occupational Category. *Employee Assistance Quarterly.* 1:25-34, 1986.

4. Foxman, Betsy, Dee W. Edington. The Accuracy of Health Risk Appraisal in Predicting Mortality. *American Journal of Public Health.* 77(8), pp. 971-974, 1987.

5. Yen, Louis Tze-ching, Dee W. Edington, Pam Witting. Associations between Health Risk Appraisal Scores and Employee Medical Claims Costs in a Manufacturing Company. *American Journal of Health Promotion.* 6:46-54, 1991.

6. Gazmararian, Julie A., Betsy Foxman, Louis Tze-ching Yen, Hall Morgenstern, Dee W. Edington. Comparing the Predictive Accuracy of the Health Risk Appraisal: The Centers for Disease Control versus the Carter Center Program. *American Journal of Public Health.* 81:1296-1301, 1991.

7. Yen, Louis Tze-ching, Dee W. Edington. Prediction of Prospective Medical Claims and Absenteeism. Costs for 1,284 Hourly Workers from a Manufacturing Company. *Journal of Occupational Medicine.* 34:428-435, 1992.

8. Edington, Dee W., Louis Yen. Is it Possible to Simultaneously Reduce Risk Factors and Excess Healthcare Costs? *American Journal of Health Promotion.* 6(6): 403-406, 1992.

9. Edington, Dee W., Louis Yen. Reliability, Validity and Effectiveness of Health Risk Appraisals. Chapter in *SPM Directory of Health Risk Appraisals.* Society of Prospective Medicine. Indianapolis, p 27-38, 1992.

10. Yen, Louis Tze-ching, Dee W. Edington, Pamela Witting. Corporate Medical Claims Cost Distribution and Factors Associated with High-Cost Status. *Journal of Occupational Medicine.* 36:505-515, 1994.

11. Conrad, Karen M., Richard Campbell, Dee W. Edington, Halley Faust, Douglas Vilnius. The Worksite Environment as a Cue to Smoking Reduction. *Research in Nursing and Health*. 19: 21-31, 1996.

12. Edington, Marilyn, Mary Ann Sharp, Kelley Vreeken, Louis Yen, Dee W. Edington. Worksite Health Program Preferences by Gender and Health Risk. *American Journal of Health Behavior*. 21 (3): 207-215, 1997.

13. Edington, Dee W., Louis Tze-ching Yen, Pamela Witting. The Financial Impact of Changes in Personal Health Practices. *Journal of Occupational and Environmental Medicine*. 39 (11): 1037-1046, 1997.

14. Musich, Shirley A., Wayne N. Burton, Dee W. Edington. Costs and Benefits of Prevention and Disease Management. *Disease Management and Health Outcomes*. 5(3): 153-166, 1999.

15. Burton, Wayne N., Daniel J. Conti, Chin-Yu Chen, Alyssa B. Schultz, Dee W. Edington. The Role of Health Risk Factors and Disease on Worker Productivity. *Journal of Occupational and Environmental Health*. 41(10): 863-877, 1999.

16. Musich, Shirley A., Deborah Napier, Dee W. Edington. The Association of Health Risks with Workers' Compensation Costs. *Journal of Occupational and Environmental Medicine*. 43(6):534-541, 2001.

17. Edington, Dee W. Emerging Research: A View from One Research Center. *American Journal of Health Promotion*. 15(5):341-349, 2001.

18. Braunstein, Alexandra, Yi Li, David Hirschland, Tim McDonald, Dee W. Edington. Internal Associations among Health-risk Factors and Risk Prevalence. *American Journal of Health Behavior*. 25(4): 407-417, 2001.

19. Yen, Louis, Marilyn Edington, Dee Edington. Changes in Health Risks among the Participants in the UAW-GM LifeSteps Health Promotion Program. *American Journal of Health Promotion*. 16(1): 7-15, 2001.

20. Park, Jin H., Dee W. Edington. A Sequential Neural Network Model for Diabetes Prediction. *Artificial Intelligence in Medicine*. 23(2001): 277-293, 2001.

21. Edington, Marilyn P., Terry Karjalainen, Dee W. Edington. The UAW-GM Health Promotion Program: Successful Outcomes. *American Association of Occupational Health Nursing Journal*. 50(1): 26-31, 2002.

22. Schultz, Alyssa B., Chifung Lu, Tracey E. Barnett, Louis Tze-ching Yen, Timothy McDonald, David Hirschland, Dee W. Edington. Influence of Participation in a Worksite Health Promotion Program on Disability Days. *Journal of Occupational and Environmental Medicine.* 44(8): 776-780, 2002.

23. Wright, Douglas W., Marshall J. Beard, Dee W. Edington. Association of Health Risks with the Cost of Time Away from Work. *Journal of Occupational and Environmental Medicine.* 44(12):1126-1134, 2002.

24. Edington, Dee W., Wayne N. Burton. Health and Productivity. Chapter in McCunney, R. J. A Practical Approach to Occupational and Environmental Medicine. 3rd Edition. Lippincott, Williams, & Wilkins. P 140-152. 2003.

25. Musich, Shirley, Timothy McDonald, David Hirschland, Dee W. Edington. Examination of Risk Status Transitions among Active Employees in a Comprehensive Worksite Health Promotion Program. *Journal of Occupational and Environmental Medicine.* 45(4):393-399, 2003.

26. Edington, Dee W., Shirley Musich. The Case for Low-Risk Maintenance. *Absolute Advantage.* 2(5):22-25, 2003.

27. Yen, Louis, Timothy McDonald, David Hirschland, Dee W. Edington. Association Between Wellness Score from a Health Risk Appraisal and Prospective Medical Claims Costs. *Journal of Occupational and Environmental Medicine.* 45(10):1049-1057, 2003.

28. Musich, Shirley, Stephanie D. Faruzzi, Chi-Fung Lu, Timothy McDonald, David Hirschland, Dee W. Edington. Pattern of Medical Charges after Quitting Smoking among Those with and without Arthritis, Allergies, or Back Pain. *American Journal of Health Promotion.* 18(2):133-142. 2003.

29. Park, Jin, Dee W. Edington. Application of a Prediction Model for Identification of Individuals at Diabetic Risk. *Methods Informatics in Medicine.* 43(3): 293-301, 2004.

30. Burton, Wayne N., Glen Pransky, Dan Conti, Chin-Yu Chen, Dee W. Edington. The Association of Medical Conditions and Presenteeism. *Journal of Occupational and Environmental Medicine.* 46(6):S38-S45. 2004.

31. Musich, Shirley A., Alyssa Schultz, Wayne N. Burton, D. W. Edington. Overview of Corporate-Sponsored Disease Management Programs. *Disease Management and Health Outcomes.* 12(5):299-326. 2004.

32. Burton, Wayne N., Chin-Yu Chen, Dan Conti, Glen Pransky, Dee W. Edington. Caregiving for Ill Dependents and Its Association with Employee Health Risks and Productivity. *Journal of Occupational and Environmental Medicine.* 46(10):1048-1056. 2004.

33. Cross, Margaret Ann. Spend Money on Healthy People: Interview with Dee W. Edington. *Managed Care.* August 2004.

34. Edington, Dee W. How Health Risk Appraisals Can Take Your Program to the Next Level. Wellness Councils of America: A WELCOA Expert Interview (Parts 1 and 2). 2004.

35. Edington, D.W. Managing Your Low-Risk Population. *Health Promotion Practitioner.* 14(1):7-8, 2005.

36. Burton, Wayne N., Chin-Yu Chen, Dan Conti, Alyssa Schultz, Glen Pransky, Dee W. Edington. The Association of Health Risks with On-the-Job Productivity. *Journal of Occupational and Environmental Medicine.* 47(8):769-777. 2005.

37. Wang, Feifei, Timothy McDonald, Laura Champagne and Dee W. Edington. Association of BMI, Physical Activity and Healthcare Utilization/Costs among Medicare Retirees. *Obesity Research.* 13(3):1450-1457, 2005.

38. Yen, Louis, Alyssa B. Schultz, Timothy McDonald, Laura Champagne, Dee W. Edington. Participation in Employer-Sponsored Wellness Programs Before and After Retirement. *American Journal of Health Behavior.* 30(1):27-38, 2006.

39. Burton, Wayne, Chin-Yu Chen, Daniel Conti, Alyssa Schultz, Dee W. Edington. The Association between Health Risk Change and Presenteeism Change. *Journal of Occupational and Environmental Medicine.* 48:252-263, 2006.

40. Lynch, Wendy, Chin-Yu Chen, Joel Bender, Dee W. Edington. Observed Attrition Rates in an Employer-Sponsored Disease management Program: A Possible New Metric. *Journal of Occupational and Environmental Medicine.* 48:447-454, 2006.

41. Edington, D.W. The Economic Value of Healthy Employees. *Business Journal of Phoenix.* Jump-start Your Company's Productivity. P. 11-13, June 2006.

42. Wang, Feifei, Tim McDonald, Joel Bender, Bonnie Reffitt, Adam Miller, Dee W. Edington. Association of Healthcare Costs with Per Unit BMI Increase. *Journal of Occupational and Environmental Medicine.* 48(7):668-674), 2006.

43. Yen, Louis, Alyssa Schultz, Elaine Schnueringer, Dee W Edington. Financial Costs Due to Excess Health Risks among Active Employees of a Utility Company. *Journal of Occupational and Environmental Medicine.* 48: 896-905, 2006.

44. Edington, Dee W. Who are the Intended Beneficiaries (Targets) of Employee Health Promotion and Wellness Programs? *North Carolina Medical Journal.* 67(6):425-427, 2006.

45. Edington, Dee W. The Pharmaceutical Industry as a Partner in the Emerging Population Healthcare System. Health Industries Research Companies. Spring 2007.

46. Petersen, Ruth, Stewart Sill, Chi-Fung Lu, Joyce Young, Dee W. Edington. Effectiveness of Employee Internet-Based Weight Management Program. *Journal of Occupational and Environmental Medicine.* 50(2):163-171, 2007.

47. Cyr, Amanda, Susan Hagen. Measurement and Quantification of Presenteeism. Letter to the Editor, *Journal and Occupational and Environmental Medicine.* 49(12):1299-1300, 2007.

48. Schultz, Alyssa B., Dee W. Edington. Employee Health and Presenteeism: A Systemic Review. *Journal of Occupational Rehabilitation.* 17(3):547-579, 2007.

49. Edington, Dee W. Working towards a Well Workforce. *Michigan Forward.* 22(6):4-4-6, 2007.

50. Petersen, Ruth, Stewart Sill, Chi-fung Lu, Joyce Young, Dee W. Edington. Effectiveness of Employee Internet-Based Weight Management Program. *Journal of Occupational and Environmental Medicine.* 50(2):163-171, 2008.

51. Edington, Dee W., Alyssa Schultz. The Total Value of Health: A Review of the Literature. *International Journal of Workplace Health Management.* 1(1):8-19, 2008.

52. Burton, Wayne N., Chin-Yu Chen, Alyssa B Schultz, Dee W. Edington. The Association between a Tiered Pharmacy Benefit Plan and Medication Usage, Health Status and Disability Absence Days. 50(10):1176-1184, 2008.

53. Burton, Wayne N., Alyssa B Schultz, Chin-Yu Chen, Dee W. Edington. The Association of Worker Productivity and Mental Health: A Review of the Literature. *International Journal of Workplace Health Management.* 1(2):78-94, 2008.

54. Pai, Chih-Wen, Dee W. Edington. Association between Intention for Change and Actual Change in Physical Activity, Smoking, and Body Weight. J*ournal of Occupational and Environmental Medicine.* 50(9):1077-10-83, 2008.

55. Burton, Wayne N., Chin-Yu Chen, Alyssa B. Schultz, Dee W. Edington. The Prevalence of Metabolic Syndrome in an Employed Population and the Impact on Health and Productivity. *Journal of Occupational and Environmental Medicine.* 50(10):1139-1148, 2008.

56. Lu, Chi-fung, Alyssa B. Schultz, Stewart Sill, Ruth Petersen, Joyce M. Young, Dee W. Edington. Effects of an Incentive-Based Online Physical Activity Intervention on Healthcare Costs. *Journal of Occupational and Environmental Medicine.* 50(11):1209-1215, 2008.

56 Readings from Others

(in Alphabetical Order)

57. Allen, Judd. Wellness Leadership: Creating supportive environments for healthier and more productive employees. Healthyculture. Burlington VT. 2008

58. Allen, Judd. Healthy Habits, Helpful Friends: How to Effectively Support Wellness Lifestyle Goals. Healthyculture. Burlington VT. 2008

59. Allen, Robert F., Shirley Linde. Lifegain. Appleton-Century-Crofts. 1981.

60. Aldana, Steven G. The Culprit & the Cure. Maple Mountain Press, Mapleton, Utah. 2005.

61. A Purchaser's Guide to Clinical Preventive Services: Moving Science into Coverage. Editors Kathryn Phillips Campbell, Andrew Lanza. National Business Group on Health. Washington D.C. 2006.

62. Blanchard, Ken, Susan Fowler Woodring. Empowerment: Achieving Peak Performance through Self-Leadership. Successories. 2007.

63. Blanchard, Ken, Paul J. Meyer, Dick Ruhe. Know Can Do: Put Your Know-How into Action. Berrett-Koehler Publisher. San Francisco. 2007

64. Blanchard, Ken, Thad Lacinak, Chuck Tompkins, Jim Ballard. Whale Done, The Power of Positive Relationships. Free Press, A Division of Simon & Schuster, New York. 2002

65. Blanchard, Kenneth, Susan Fowler, Lawrence Hawkins. Self-Leadership and the One Minute Manager. HarperCollins, 2005.

66. Blanchard, Kenneth, Dee Edington, Marjorie Blanchard. The One Minute Manager Balances Work and Life. William Morrow, NY. 1999.

67. Blanchard, Ken. Leading at a Higher Level. Prentice Hall, NJ 2007

68. Blanchard, Marjorie, Mark Tager. Working Well: Managing for Health & High Performance. Simon and Schuster, 1985.

69. Bloom, D.E., D. Canning. The Health and Wealth of Nations. *Science.* 287(5456):1207-1209. 2000.

70. Bunn, William. Continuing Editorials. *Journal of Health & Productivity.* 1(1):1. 2006

71. Burton, Wayne, P. W. Brandt-Rauf. Health and Productivity. A Review of the State-of-the-Art and Implications for Occupational and Environmental Medicine. *Journal of Italian Medicine and Laboratory Ergonomics.* 30(1): 15-29. 2008.

72. Chapman, Larry. Enhancing Consumer Health skills Through Worksite Health Promotion. *American Journal of Health Promotion: The Art of Health Promotion.* 22(5):1-12. 2008.

73. Chenoweth, David H. Worksite Health Promotion. Second Edition. Human Kinetics, Champaign IL. 2007

74. Collins, James. Good to Great: Why Some Companies Make the Leap and Others Don't. HarperCollins. New York. 2001

75. Collins, J.J., C. M. Baase, C. E. Sharda, R. Z. Ozminkowski, S. Nicholson, G. M. Billotti, R. S. Turpin, M. Olson, M. L. Berger. The assessment of chronic health conditions on work performance, absence and total economic impact for employers. *Journal of Occupational and Environmental Medicine.* 47:547-57. 2005.

76. Crossing the Quality Chasm: A New Health System for the 21st Century, Committee on the Quality of Healthcare in America. Institute of Medicine. National Academy of Sciences. 2000.

77. Darling, Helen. Healthcare 2009: Issues and Challenges. *Human Resource Executive.* November 19, 2008.

78. Deal, Terrence E., Allan A. Kennedy. Corporate Cultures. Addison-Wesley. Reading, MA. 1982.

79. Employer Health Asset Management: A Roadmap for Improving the Health of Your Employees and Your Organization. Change Agent Work Group. 2009.

80. Freudenheim, Milt. Building better Bodies. *New York Times.* October 1, 2008. p H1, H6.

81. Gladwell, Malcolm. The Tipping Point. How Little Things Can Make a Dig Difference. Little, Brown and Company. New York. 2000.

82. Goetzel, R. Z., S. R. Long, R. J. Ozminkowski, K. Hawkins, S. Wang, W. Lynch. Health, Absence, Disability, and Presenteeism Cost Estimates of Certain Physical and Mental Health Conditions Affecting U.S. Employers. *Journal of Occupational and Environmental Medicine.* 46:398-412. 2004.

83. Golaszewski, Thomas, Judd Allen, Dee W. Edington. The Role of the Environment in Health Management Programs. *American Journal of Health Promotion: The Art of Health Promotion.* 22(4):1-10, 2008.

84. Health & Work Productivity. Edited by Ronald C. Kessler and Paul E. Stang. University of Chicago Press. 2006.

85. Holland, John H. Emergence: From Chaos to Order. Perseus Books 1998.

86. Hamel, Gary, C. K. Prahalad. Competing for the Future. Harvard Business School Press. 1994.

87. Heussner, Steve. Fit to Succeed. MH Publishing LLC. Dallas, TX 2008.

88. Heng, Henry H. Q. The Conflict between Complex Systems and Reductionism. Commentary. *Journal of the American Medical Association.* 300(13):1580-1581, 2008.

89. Hunnicutt, David. Developing a Data Dashboard: The Art and Science of Making Sense. Absolute Advantage. Wellness Councils of America. 6(4): 34-39. 2007.

90. Integrating Employee Health: A Model Program for NASA. Institute of Medicine, National Academy of Sciences. 2005

91. Leading by Example. Improving the Bottom Line through a High Performance, Less Costly Workforce CEOs on the Business Case for Worksite Health Promotion. Copyright © Partnership for Prevention ® 2005. This publication may be downloaded free of charge on Partnerships Web site, www.prevent.org/LBE

92. Leading by Example. Leading Practices for Employee Health Management. Copyright © Partnership for Prevention ® 2007. This publication may be downloaded free of charge on Partnerships Web site, www.prevent.org/LBE.

93. Lerner D., S. H. Allaire, S. T. Reisine. Work Disability Resulting from Chronic Health Conditions. *Journal of Occupational and Environmental Medicine.* 2005;47:253-264.

94. Loepkke, Ronald, Sean Nicholson, Michael Taitel, Mathew Sweeney, Vince Haufle, Ronald C. Kessler. The Impact of an Integrated Population Health Enhancement and Disease Management Program on Employee Health Risk, Health Conditions, and Productivity. *Population Health Management.* 11(6):287-296. 2008.

95. Lynch, Wendy. Aligning Incentives, Information and Choice. Health and Human Capital Foundation. Cheyenne, WY. 2008

96. Mahoney, Jack, David Hom. Total Value Total Return. GlaxoSmithKline. PA. 2006.

97. Mirvis, David M., David E. Bloom. Population Health and Economic Development in the United States. *Journal of the American Medical Association.* 300(1):93-95, 2008.

98. Musich, Shirley, Timothy McDonald, Larry S. Chapman. Health promotion Strategies for the "Boomer" Generation: Wellness for the Mature Worker. *American Journal of Health Promotion: The Art of Health Promotion.* 23(3):1-12. 2009.

99. O'Donnell, Michael. Health Promotion in the Workplace. Third Edition. Delmar Thompson Learning., Albany, NY. 2002.

100. Ozminkowski, Ronald J., Ron Z. Goetzel, Feifei Wang, Teresa B. Gibson, David Shechter, Shirley Musich, Joel Bender, Dee W. Edington. The Savings Gained From Participation in Health Promotion Programs for Medicare Beneficiaries. *Journal of Occupational and Environmental Medicine.* 48(11):1125-1132, 2006.

101. Peters, Tom. Thriving on Chaos: A Handbook for Management Revolution. Alfred A. Knopf, Inc. 1987

102. Porter, Michael E., Elizabeth Olmsted Teisberg. How Physicians Can Change the future of Healthcare. *Journal of the American Medical Association.* 297:1103-1111. 2007.

103. Pfeiffer, George, Judith Webster. Workcare: a working person's guide to life balance. The Workcare Group, 3rd Edition. 2001,

104. Pritchett, Price. The Unfolding. Pritchett. Dallas. 2006.

105. Pelletier, Kenneth R. Sound Mind, Sound Body: A New Model for Lifelong Health. Simon & Schuster. New York. 1994.

106. Pelletier, Kenneth R. Healthy People in Unhealthy Workplaces: Stress and Fitness at Work. Delacorne Press. New York. 1984.

107. Powell, Don. Healthier at Home: The Proven Guide to Self-Care & Being a Wise Health Consumer. American Institute of Preventive Medicine. Farmington Hills, MI. 2007.

108. Quinn, Robert E. Deep Change: Discovering the Leader Within. Jossey-Bass Publishers, San Francisco. 1996.

109. Rearick, David, Good Health is Good Business: an Implementation Guide for Corporate Wellness. Strategic Benefit Solutions. Atlanta. 2007.

110. Rosen, Robert H. Just Enough Anxiety: The Hidden Driver of Business Success. Penguin Group. New York. 2008

111. Fries, James F., Vickery, Donald M. Take Care of Yourself. Sixth Edition. Addison Wesley. New York. 1994.

112. Worksite Wellness Program Keeps Employees Healthy. Research Brief. Center for Health Improvement. Sacramento, July 2008.

Current and Past UM-HMRC Consortium Members

The following companies are members (past or current) of the UM-HMRC Corporate Consortium. The Consortium exists to allow companies with like interests in Health Management to meet together for one day in Ann Arbor during the first or second week in December. There are no membership fees, the only requirement is that they are committed to a long-term investment in the health and productivity of their company and their employees and the UM-HMRC works in partnership with them to measure, evaluate and provide decision support metrics.

1. Affinity Health Plan
2. Allegiance Health System
3. Australian Health Management Corporation
4. AutoNation
5. Caterpillar, Inc.
6. Crown Equipment
7. Cuyahoga Community College
8. Delphi Automotive
9. Florida Power & Light
10. Ford Motor Company
11. General Motors
12. JP Morgan Chase
13. Kellogg Corporation
14. Medical Mutual of Ohio
15. Navistar
16. Progressive Corporation
17. Southern Company/Gulf Power
18. Southwest Michigan Healthcare Coalition
19. Steelcase Corporation
20. St Luke's Health System
21. United Auto Workers-Ford
22. United Auto Workers-General Motors
23. University of Missouri
24. U.S. Steel
25. We Energies
26. Wisconsin Education Association Trust